◆ **Based on Nobel Prize Science** ◆

THE
WELLNESS
SOLUTION

◆

By
Edward A. Taub, M.D., F.A.A.P.
Ferid Murad, M.D., Ph.D.
David Oliphant

The contents of this book are a reflection of the authors' philosophy, beliefs and clinical experience. The ideas, suggestions, and procedures contained in the book are not intended to be a substitute for consultation with your own physician before beginning any new regimen.

World Almanac Library of Wellness books are published by

World Almanac Library
An imprint of
Gareth Stevens Inc.
330 W. Olive Street
Milwaukee, WI 53212

A co-publishing venture with
Taub-Murad-Oliphant Medical Research Associates, LLC
284 Racebrook Road
Orange, CT 06477

Photo credits:
Dr. Taub's photo by Siegfried Hopf
David Oliphant's photo by Stuart Walls of Woodstock Studios

Library of Congress Cataloging-in-Publication Data

Taub, Edward A.
The wellness solution / by Edward A. Taub, Ferid Murad, David Oliphant.
p. cm.
Includes bibliographical references and index.
ISBN-13: 978-0-8368-8163-9
ISBN-10: 0-8368-8163-X
1. Health. 2. Nutrition. 3. Exercise. I. Murad, Ferid. II. Oliphant, David, 1935- III. Title.
RA776.T257 2007
613—dc22
2006036307

First Printing: December 2006
10 9 8 7 6 5 4 3 2 1

Printed in the United States of America

Cover Design by Deborah Kalman

"To Our Mothers And Wives."

TABLE OF CONTENTS

PART FIVE

PERSONAL EVALUATION *205*

PART SIX

WRAPPING UP *214*

FOREWORD

Surely the greatest miracle we all cherish is the miracle of life itself. Now, two extraordinarily accomplished medical doctors have identified the Nitric Oxide molecule as the actual "Spark of Life." Nitric Oxide is an invisible gas that protects our greatest asset—our health. Boosting this invisible gas in your body is as important to your health and well-being as the oxygen you breathe. This is the basis for *The Wellness Solution*.

My name is David Oliphant, and I am the publisher and co-author of *The Wellness Solution*. I am privileged to publish this book about a remarkable discovery that gives you a new reason to lead a healthier lifestyle. My role is to present the doctors' groundbreaking work in a way that will help you understand how you can determine your own health destiny. If *The Wellness Solution* had been written just for doctors, instead of for the countless millions of people who want to preserve their health and well-being, the book might have been appropriately called *The Molecular Biology of Wellness*.

The discovery of the connection between Nitric Oxide and your health is simple to understand. The major reason we feel better when we eat healthfully, manage our weight, drink appropriate amounts of water, take a scientifically balanced vitamin and mineral nutritional system, exercise regularly, refrain from smoking, and manage our stress (which includes being a good person), is because all these things help boost the Nitric Oxide in our bodies! This significant discovery can support a healthy life and will allow you to age with less pain and suffering than is usually associated with getting older. . . . That's *The Wellness Solution.*

One of my proudest accomplishments in life is being a part of the publishing industry for more than 40 years. My life began in the South Bronx. I was a street kid who at the age of 17 went on to become a pitcher in the minor leagues for the New York Yankees and the Los Angeles Dodgers. Baseball afforded me the opportunity to pursue my college education. I went from throwing a great fastball to presenting great books in ways that people could easily understand and enjoy.

Those who remember the world-famous "Illustrated Classics" know my work, which consisted of translating great literature into exciting and easy-to-read books, supported by fabulous illustrations that helped millions of people discover and understand the wonderful world of the great classics.

Under my direction, over 100 million copies of these great books were printed and sold, including those by such immortal authors as Herman Melville, Robert Louis Stevenson, Jules Verne, Stephen Crane, Samuel Clemens, Emily Brontë, Jack London, Richard Dana, Alexander Dumas, H.G. Wells, and William Shakespeare. The list goes on and on, but the point I want to make here is that my goal was to present great books by outstanding minds in ways that would be understandable to virtually everyone. I believe this has been accomplished with *The Wellness Solution.*

One thing I have learned in my publishing career is that the rules never really change! Every publisher is always looking for "the next big book," and it is my honor to write this foreword, because *The Wellness Solution* is the next big book.

Another proud accomplishment was being the president of Connecticut's Fairfield County Chapter of the Leukemia & Lymphoma Society for more than eight years, while also serving on its board of trustees for over 30 years as a volunteer. My main mission in life has always been to help people, and I believe this book will help millions and millions of people.

So, how could one more health book make me this excited? Aren't bookstore shelves filled with plenty of advice on health? After working with these two brilliant doctors on this book, I can honestly tell you that their incredible knowledge about how you can stay healthy and live longer, with less pain and suffering, is worthy of being worldwide headline news!

Edward A.Taub, M.D., has been a board-certified pediatrician and a family doctor for over 40 years and is truly a gift to humanity. He spends more than half his life researching the latest medical information to stay up-to-date for his patients' well-being. That type of dedication is almost unheard of in the practice of medicine today. As QVC's "Wellness Medical Doctor," he probably has the largest medical practice in the world. I consider Dr. Taub "America's Wellness Medical Doctor."

Ferid Murad, M.D., Ph.D., is also an extraordinary and dedicated doctor. His research is the basis for the science in this book. **He shared the 1998 Nobel Prize in Medicine for his research leading to the discovery that Nitric Oxide is the body's "signaling molecule."** This means that NO, the chemical name for Nitric Oxide, helps determine your body's functions, including your ability to stay healthy by reducing the risk of degenerative diseases. Can you imagine anything more important than this? I certainly can't! Dr. Murad also received the Albert Lasker Award for Basic Medical Research—the most prestigious medical science award in the United States—for *"having advanced the fundamental understanding of biochemical mechanisms in cells."*

As I mentioned earlier, these two incredibly gifted doctors have identified the Nitric Oxide molecule as the Spark of Life. Nitric Oxide is truly a miracle molecule which provides the missing link for preserving health. This is the molecular basis for *The Wellness Solution*. The strategy of boosting production of Nitric Oxide in the entire body, naturally, without drugs, through *The Wellness Solution* has never been presented to the public before—*that's why I am so excited!*

The doctors and I first got together in Houston, Texas, where Dr. Murad is the director of the Institute of Molecular Medicine and the chairman of the University of Texas Medical School Department of Integrative Biology and Pharmacology. There, we discussed writing a book together about how to boost NO in the body and the amazing benefits of doing so. I was mesmerized by the challenge of how I could possibly take the incredible knowledge from these two gifted doctors and translate it onto the printed page in a way that we could all relate to and understand. Both Drs. Taub and Murad looked at me, laughed, and said, "Dave, that's your job! You've done it before, so let's go for it!" I accepted the challenge.

As both publisher and co-author, my role was to put the doctors' voices together so they could speak as one to the countless millions of people all over the world who need practical and reliable guidance to help stem the rising tide of chronic degenerative diseases and the suffering these illnesses cause. I decided to make their awesome medical breakthrough both motivational and easy to understand so that no one who reads the book can ignore it.

Let's face it: Health education should not end with merely accumulating information. It should transform our habits, our characters, and our aspirations as well. Indeed, once you glimpse through the self-evident truths in our book, I predict you won't be able to turn your back on *The Wellness Solution.*

Previously, I had written a book with Dr. Lawrence B. Slobody, former president of New York Medical College, called *The Golden Years.* He believed the human body was built to last 115 years! If you had read that statement 50 years ago, you probably would have thought that the good doctor was insane, and reading it today, you probably think he was being a little overly optimistic. Well, what do you think life expectancy will be in another 25 years from now? Probably a whole lot closer to age 115 than it was 50 years ago!

To repeat . . . boosting your body's Nitric Oxide is essential, because it's as important as the oxygen you breathe, and you can't live without it! Let me give you another example. . . . If you were having a hard time breathing because you were not getting enough oxygen in your blood, your doctor might prescribe oxygen in a small tank that could be carried around with you. Someday, that same type of help will probably be available for Nitric Oxide gas as well.

But why wait? Almost 100,000 research studies on Nitric Oxide have been published since Dr. Murad won the Nobel Prize in Medicine. New ways of boosting lifesaving Nitric Oxide in your body are just now being discovered by the drug industry, and projections are that it will soon become a hundred-billion-dollar-per-year industry. (By the way, Viagra was the first blockbuster drug based on Dr. Murad's research.)

But again, why wait? Why not begin with the most natural and noninvasive way to boost Nitric Oxide in your body . . . *The Wellness Solution.*

I am thankful to Drs. Taub and Murad for allowing me the opportunity to help them get their message out to the world through this book. It's a call to action by two very wise and compassionate physicians who care deeply about humankind, patients, and their profession.

Please read on!

Always remember, your health is your most precious asset.

David Oliphant,
Publisher/Co-author

INTRODUCTION

THE ANSWER IS NO . . . WHICH REALLY IS YES!

The time is right and the need is great for a genuine medical revolution to help you stay healthy and feel well. Do you think you are ready for it? You probably think you are, but your mind may not be as ready as you think.

In fact, the minds of most Americans have been programmed by the disease-care industry to feel sick in order to get you to take the newest and most expensive drugs, often for diseases you would not know about unless you watched the drug commercials on television. The United States Office of Management and Budget recently estimated that medical care will use up 20 percent of every dollar spent by 2015. This is very disheartening and confusing because we already spend more money on medical care in America than the gross national product of most nations in the world *combined!*

Think about what a world we live in! The leading *causes of deaths* in the United States are chronic degenerative diseases, especially heart disease, cancer, and stroke. Remarkably, the leading *preventable causes of deaths* in the United States are smoking, obesity, and the negative side effects of prescription drugs. So why aren't we doing something about this? It makes no sense.

Maybe the reason we aren't doing something is because we have been searching for answers in the wrong places. This book, written by two dedicated medical doctors and a uniquely experienced publisher, provides a revolutionary answer.

The answer to good health is NO . . . which really means yes. We need to explain that NO, as used throughout this book, refers specifically to the chemical symbol for the Nitric Oxide molecule. NO does not refer to the word no. NO, a chemical symbol, is pronounced by saying each letter: N followed by O (en-owe). By the way, Nitric Oxide is not the same thing as "laughing gas," which some dentists use. That's *nitrous* oxide.

Why does NO translate to yes? Because Dr. Ferid Murad's Nobel Prize–winning research can help solve the most glaring health problem of our time, which is the fact that most Americans are now living to a much older age and are consequently developing more chronic degenerative diseases. Half of all baby boomers will have at least one chronic degenerative disease by the time they are 65 years old, and most will probably go on to develop two or three chronic degenerative diseases. As a matter of fact 20 percent of Americans over the age of 65 have five or more chronic degenerative diseases. So, in spite of spending so much money to maintain our health, we are getting sicker for longer with diseases of the heart, blood vessels, blood, brain, nerves, stomach, liver, intestines, kidneys, bladder, genital organs, bones, and joints. Clearly, we need an effective answer to aging in our society that will make the process worth *living* for!

This book provides the vision as well as the solution that *does* make age worth living for. By reading on, you will prepare your mind for the new and factual information that heralds a medical revolution based on NO. This is a genuine paradigm discovery that will literally amaze you.

Are there other answers? Of course, but be aware of what we already touched upon. Our minds are being programmed by a powerful disease-care industry.

What about more drugs, surgical procedures, and diagnostic tests? How can those be the answer when we Americans are already the most over-medicated, over-hospitalized, over-radiated, and over-tested people on our entire planet?

What about a stronger managed health care industry? How can that be the answer when most of the industry's efforts to contain health costs have led to even higher costs as it tries to achieve greater profits?

What about socialized medicine, or virtually free medical care for everyone? How can that be the answer when it must ultimately be paid for with higher taxes and more bureaucracy, which eventually keep patients away from needed medical care?

What about merely providing information on preventive medicine so people will take better care of themselves and stay healthier in the first place? That's a partial answer, but not a very realistic one, since most Americans already know that unhealthy lifestyles are the major cause of disease, disability, and death. Yet so many Americans still smoke, eat in excess, and refuse to exercise regularly.

It all boils down to the fact that the answer is NO and *The Wellness Solution.* NO is the scientific basis for *The Wellness Solution*, which helps build the physical, psychological, and spiritual strengths required for health and well-being.

- *Physical* strength is necessary to slow down the disease process caused by the ever-present force called entropy, which makes our cells become sick and eventually die.

- *Psychological* strength is needed to combat our feelings of wanting to "give up" on our healthful commitments because we think good health is "too difficult to achieve" or that "it's too late to change."

- *Spiritual* strength, which grows as we develop reverence for life, is required for us to feel worthy of making and keeping our commitments to take charge of our own health destiny.

So, the answer is NO because NO helps slow down the force of entropy and helps control stress by generating the healthy attitude that we truly can help ourselves. This is a relatively foreign concept because modern medicine is based almost entirely on efforts to repair the body rather than stimulate its natural will to be well. Modern medicine has neglected the age-old concept that health is largely determined by our own personal responsibility, self-value, and reverence for life.

We need to stimulate our internal healing strengths, which *The Wellness Solution* can do for us. Can you think of anything more valuable than your health? No matter how wealthy or successful you are, even the slightest headache, earache, sore throat, or even something as simple as a splinter in your finger or a hair in your eye can make you feel very uncomfortable and out of balance. More serious symptoms of illness or disease can permanently replace any joy in your life with total sadness. Being healthy is the most precious gift we can give ourselves. This is why unleashing the power of NO by following *The Wellness Solution* can bring us such wonderful benefits.

Even though the health care system in America is flawed, we are convinced that the nobility of medicine remains. We are honored to serve as your guides while traveling the path to wellness. The story we tell in this book will come from one voice representing three co-authors. At times the voice is mostly Dr. Ferid Murad's. Other times the voice is mostly Dr. Edward Taub's. At certain times, the voice is mostly David Oliphant's. But always, and at all times, we speak to every reader who wants to know now what we usually learn only when we are much older.

Dr. Murad was awarded the 1998 Nobel Prize in Medicine for his research leading to the remarkable discovery that *Nitric Oxide is the body's signaling molecule.* That means that NO determines your body's functions, including its ability to stay healthy and recover from disease. Therefore, we have identified NO as the Spark of Life and *The Wellness Solution* as your prescription for a healthier, longer life. The following pages will give you a clearer understanding of NO and teach you, through *The Wellness Solution*, how to boost NO in your body. We regard this book as one of our most memorable contributions to humanity.

PART ONE

NITRIC OXIDE (NO) AND ENDOTHELIAL HEALTH

A New Biologic Principle

For everything there is a season, and a time for every matter under heaven: a time to be born, and a time to die . . . a time to break down, and a time to build up.
—Ecclesiastes

We have identified the human body's Spark of Life. Just as importantly, we have identified *The Wellness Solution* as a safe, effective way to ignite that Spark of Life.

Would you believe the Spark of Life is a simple gas, capable of transmitting a signal to live or die to our cells, tissues, and organs? And it's not oxygen. Instead, it's a more primitive, unstable molecule, and perhaps the oldest life-supporting molecule to appear on Earth. It's an invisible gas called Nitric Oxide. Again, the chemical name for Nitric Oxide is NO.

Dr. Ferid Murad shared the 1998 Nobel Prize in Medicine with Dr. Robert F. Furchgott and Dr. Louis J. Ignarro for the world-shaking discovery that the NO molecule is a "signaling molecule" in the body. The notion of a gas being able to send signals between cells all over the body was a groundbreaking new concept. Put simply, NO molecules can tell the body to stay well, repair itself, or die.

The fact that NO is a gas makes Dr. Murad's discovery even more exciting in terms of preserving our health. Why? This gas is not restricted in its travels through the body by the barrier membranes surrounding our cells. Instead, NO can move freely, permeating the membranes to deliver signals to and from all parts of the body to help preserve its health. Just think of NO as being like an invisible mist traveling in an uninhibited manner through the cells, tissues, and organs of your body. What a dramatic discovery!

A sufficient amount of NO signals the cells of the heart, blood vessels, brain, nerves, stomach, liver, intestines, immune system, bones, joints, bladder, and sex organs to stay healthy and function well. This is the healing force scientists call homeostasis. On the other hand, NO gas, by its absence or in an insufficient quantity, signals our cells, tissues, and organs to degenerate. This is part of the force scientists call entropy, which causes everything in nature to eventually fall apart.

So far, the most widespread application of Dr. Murad's Nobel Prize–winning research has been the development of Viagra and Viagra-like drugs to help the penis achieve an erection. The wildly popular Viagra was designed to increase the effect of NO, which makes blood vessels wider by relaxing the smooth muscles in their walls. Viagra helps trigger erections by relaxing blood vessels in the penis so it can accommodate more blood. Is there more to NO than Viagra? *Of course there is.* NO ensures blood flow to the entire body, and *The Wellness Solution* is the natural, noninvasive way to make it happen.

Valentin Fuster, M.D., Ph.D., the president of the American Heart Association in 1998, declared, "The discovery of Nitric Oxide and its function is one of the most important in the history of cardiovascular medicine."

We agree, which is why we feel honored to present *The Wellness Solution* to help you reduce your risk of cardiovascular disease, as well as other chronic degenerative diseases throughout the body. Simply stated, **people with high levels of NO in their bodies are generally healthier than people who have low levels of NO in their bodies.**

How big a difference can this make to you? Very big! As you read on, you'll learn why NO is equivalent to your body's own natural nitroglycerin—the classic heart medicine doctors use to treat chest pain and prevent heart attacks. Like nitroglycerin, NO can signal an explosion of good health. Dr. Murad's Nobel Prize–winning research led to the discovery that nitroglycerin works by stimulating production of NO in the coronary arteries, which relaxes and widens the vessels and in turn allows oxygen-enriched blood to flow through those arteries to nourish the heart. But before we go any further, we need to explain some basic chemistry and anatomy. We are confident we can make it easy to understand.

What Exactly Is NO?

NO is an unstable, "free-radical" molecule that helps relax and widen our blood vessels to allow delivery of oxygen to virtually every cell and organ in the body. Most of the NO in your body is produced by a thin layer of cells called the endothelium, which coats the insides of your blood vessels. Our lung cells, white blood cells, and the nerve cells of your brain also produce NO. To a lesser extent, most other cells of the body may also produce NO.

How unstable are NO molecules? Very! They generally last only two to three seconds in the body. NO is also a very simple molecule—it consists of just one atom of nitrogen bound to one atom of oxygen. Compared with all the incredibly complex molecules in the body, the NO molecule is simplicity itself . . . as well as a very good free radical.

We usually think of free-radical molecules as being "bad" for our health, but NO is a "good" free radical. It's almost like the fact that there is "good" cholesterol (HDL) and "bad" cholesterol (LDL).

So, NO is a friendly free radical—and a life-saving one at that! By helping to ensure blood flow to all the cells in your body, NO preserves heart health, brain health, joint health, skin health, lung health, liver health, kidney health, immune system health, sexual health, hormonal health—and much more. Basically, NO signals your cells to live longer and stay healthy. At the deepest molecular level, NO encourages homeostasis and regulates entropy. In a sense, it provides scientific substance for the quote from Ecclesiastes about "a time to break down and a time to build up." It's easy to understand why the goal of *The Wellness Solution* is boosting the levels of NO in our bodies.

As an unstable free radical, NO bonds with other molecules in the body, particularly other free radicals that result from our living in an oxygen atmosphere and from the ways we metabolize nutrients to produce the energy we require. Obviously, this ongoing chemical process decreases the level of NO in your body, so it must be put back in balance. You need to encourage your body's healthy NO-producing cells and the continuous production of NO molecules.

Just to clarify: A stable molecule consists of one or more atoms bound together with paired electrons. But a free-radical molecule has an unpaired electron that drives it to search for other molecules and snatch away their electrons. Of course, that leaves the other molecules unstable. Damage occurs in the body when those other molecules are in the heart, brain, joints, skin, lungs, liver, and elsewhere. This chemical process of snatching away electrons is called oxidation, which is the scientific term for rust!

Just as it is in our cars and in our homes, rust in our bodies is usually a sign of aging and deterioration. But instead of calling this process rust, we choose to call it degeneration and disease. Now you can truly begin understanding what chronic degenerative diseases in all parts of the body really mean. . . . *It's rust.*

Oxidation reduces the amount of NO in the body. Imagine all the NO-producing cells lining the insides of blood vessels as the cells rust away . . . then think about all the NO molecules that are still being produced. Imagine them as they are destroyed by renegade molecules that are snatching their electrons. It's not a pretty picture, and neither is the result, which is the current epidemic of chronic degenerative diseases in all parts of the body.

Some of the culprits that increase these electron-snatching thieves in the body are stress, obesity, cigarette smoke, pollution, pesticides, contaminants, radiation, and unhealthful food. It is estimated that in these modern times all our cells experience many thousands of destructive free-radical "hits" every minute. However, remember that NO is the exception. So, we hope you get it. . . . We must keep NO levels in our bodies as high as possible and take steps to protect our bodies from free radicals that cause disease. *The Wellness Solution* will help you do that.

What Exactly Is the Endothelium?

The endothelium is a very thin layer of cells lining the inside of our blood vessels. Endothelial cells are responsible for manufacturing most of our NO. How thin is the endothelium? The layer of cells lining our blood vessels is only one cell thick. That's amazing when we consider it is the source of the Spark of Life.

What's also amazing is that at one time, the endothelium was thought to be just a fine layer of inactive cells. However, thanks largely to Dr. Murad's research, we now know the endothelium is extremely active and has numerous functions, including increasing the width of our blood vessels by producing NO.

It's important to note that endothelial dysfunction (a less-than-healthy endothelium) is a major cause of chronic degenerative diseases, especially of the heart and blood vessels. However, the good news is that endothelial dysfunction can be reversed.

Again, because NO is a gas, it is able to penetrate cell membranes to regulate the function of neighboring cells as well as distant cells. It's like an airplane flying unimpeded through a dense cloud. The endothelium produces puffs or sparks of NO that exist for only a few seconds. . . . That's one of the reasons we call NO the Spark of Life. This is an entirely new principle for understanding how to preserve health and balance in the body. Let's continue.

The human vascular system is so extensive that if our blood vessels were somehow lined up end to end, they would be over 100,000 miles long! Now we know just how delicately the endothelium regulates these vessels through its production of NO. The signaling molecule relaxes and widens our blood vessels, thereby ensuring proper blood flow and the delivery of life-giving oxygen and nutrients to all parts of our bodies.

Although only one cell thick, the endothelial layer that lines the inside of our blood vessels has the surface area of about eight tennis courts. In a sense, the endothelium is a vital organ, just like the brain, lungs, pancreas, and liver. Not only that, but if you could somehow collect all the cells, they would weigh over 5 pounds and be one of the heaviest organs in the human body! (Compare that with the brain and liver. Each of those organs weighs about 3 pounds.)

Dr. Murad discovered nitroglycerin works by releasing puffs of NO molecules, which cause the walls of the coronary arteries to relax and widen. It is the same with the rest of the body. The most obvious result of the relaxing and widening process is that it regulates blood pressure, which directly affects the heart. If blood vessels are narrow, blood pressure is increased, which causes the heart to work harder to pump blood. Healthy endothelial cells producing sufficient NO also help decrease blood clots in the vessels.

NO even reduces the stickiness of blood clots once they've formed, which is a major factor in determining whether the clots will attach to the inner walls of the vessels, causing heart attacks and strokes. NO probably also decreases the formation of atherosclerotic plaque. Finally, NO helps regulate the movement of blood cells through capillary walls to support immunity, tissue repair, infection control, and general healing.

To repeat, endothelial dysfunction, which means less-than-good health in the delicate lining inside the blood vessels and therefore less NO, is a major cause of chronic degenerative disease throughout the body.

Natural Discoveries with Real Results

Did nitroglycerin act via release of Nitric Oxide? Dr.
Ferid Murad bubbled Nitric Oxide gas through tissue.
Cyclic GMP increased! A new mode of drug action had
been discovered!

—Inscription accompanying the
Nobel Prize in Medicine, 1998

Would you believe that nitroglycerin has been used for almost 150 years as both an explosive and a heart medicine?

Alfred Nobel's father was an engineer in Sweden who built bridges and buildings, and constantly experimented with different ways of blasting away rocks. Alfred Nobel thought he could help his father by making nitroglycerin into a safe explosive—at that time, most people considered nitroglycerin much too dangerous to be of any practical value. The problem was that nitroglycerin would explode in an unpredictable manner when subjected to heat or pressure.

In fact, Alfred Nobel's initial experiments with nitroglycerin killed several coworkers, including his younger brother, Emil. As a result, Swedish authorities banned further experiments within Stockholm's city limits. In response, Alfred moved his laboratory to a barge on a lake to conduct his experiments in relative safety—at least for the townsfolk.

Through his experimentation, Alfred discovered that mixing nitroglycerin liquid with fine sand would turn the liquid into paste, which could then be shaped into rods that could be placed into drilling holes and somewhat more safely be ignited to explode. Alfred Nobel named his discovery dynamite and received a patent for it in 1866. He also invented fuses and detonating caps for the dynamite, creating such a demand in the construction industry that he became one of the wealthiest men in Europe. Through his will, he established the Nobel Foundation, which awards the Nobel Prize in Medicine for discoveries that bestow the greatest benefits for mankind.

Alfred Nobel suffered greatly with angina pectoris, which is chest pain due to constriction or obstruction of the coronary arteries that deliver oxygen to the heart muscles. This often leads to death of some heart muscles, which we then call a heart attack or myocardial infarction. Coincidentally, Alfred Nobel's doctors told him to take nitroglycerin, the active ingredient in his dynamite, to relieve the pain and anxiety of his angina pectoris. The inventor wrote to a friend, "It sounds like the irony of fate that I have been prescribed nitroglycerin, internally."

In another irony of fate, 100 years later, Dr. Murad's curiosity about why nitroglycerin helps so many patients with coronary artery disease led him to the discovery that it stimulates the production of NO, which relaxes the coronary arteries and allows blood to flow more freely to deliver life-saving oxygen to the heart.

Thanks to Dr. Murad's discovery, we now know how our oldest, and still one of our most important, heart medicine works. NO is like your body's natural nitroglycerin! This is a new concept in molecular biology and a major basis for molecular medicine, which is a dynamic new science.

As director of the Institute of Molecular Medicine for the Prevention of Human Diseases in Houston, Texas, Dr. Murad now helps to focus the efforts of many distinguished scientists from all over the world on how to use this knowledge for developing new strategies for disease. The researchers are totally dedicated to the mission of the institute, which is:

> To conduct disease-oriented basic research, to make clear the cellular and molecular mechanisms underlying human diseases and to use this newly gained knowledge for the rational design of methods of treatment and, wherever possible, create strategies for the prevention of disease. Disease prevention will be the goal of medicine in the 21st century. It will save lives, reduce human suffering, and maintain the quality of life.

Most Americans, especially as they age, simply do not have sufficient amounts of NO in their bodies. Why? Because people who smoke, who are obese, who don't exercise, or who are chronically stressed probably have endothelial dysfunction. If we also count the people who have high cholesterol, atherosclerosis, hypertension, or diabetes, then the list adds up to most Americans. Fortunately, the endothelium has remarkable recuperative power. As you read on, you will learn how to ignite and detonate that power—just like Alfred Nobel did.

This is fairly complicated, but it's the basis for Dr. Murad's Nobel Prize in Medicine, so it's a worthwhile chemistry lesson to spend a few moments reading. . . .

Many of the effects of NO occur because NO stimulates the formation of another messenger molecule that's called cyclic guanosine monophosphate, or cyclic GNP. One of the effects of cyclic GNP in our blood vessels is to regulate the contractile protein machinery. This leads to the relaxation and dilation (widening) of our blood vessels. The popular drug Viagra, and similar products, inhibits the metabolism and the inactivation of cyclic GNP. Thus, drugs such as Viagra enhance the effects of NO. The effects of NO on the relaxation of blood vessels in the penis are increased with these drugs to achieve and maintain erection. However, these drugs can be associated with toxicity in some patients taking nitroglycerin or related drugs.

Boosting Nitric Oxide Production

A healthy lifestyle helps boost NO in your body. The kind of lifestyle that's needed is one which includes healthful nutrition, weight management, drinking adequate amounts of water, a medically responsible vitamin and mineral nutritional system, a no-smoking commitment, and stress management, which includes being a good person. So does working with your physician to control high cholesterol, atherosclerosis, hypertension, and diabetes. All of this can have an extremely positive impact on NO production. As a matter of fact, recent studies indicate that the vast majority of the 650,000 new heart attacks occurring each year could be prevented or delayed for decades!

The most effective way to boost NO is to support your endothelial health by utilizing the information we've shared with you, which is worth repeating over and over, because its elements are so simple yet so powerful: healthy nutrition, weight management, adequate amounts of water, scientifically balanced nutritional supplements, no smoking, and stress management, which includes being a good person.

Nutritional supplements, especially antioxidants, provide a form of additional health insurance, because the body uses the ingredients to help manufacture and sustain healthy levels of NO. In situations involving arterial inflammation, high blood pressure, diabetes, tobacco use, and the like, the endothelium becomes so dysfunctional that the vitamins and minerals we ingest from our foods alone may not be sufficient to produce a healthy amount of NO. For example, a fresh apple slice eventually turns brown when its molecules are exposed to the free-radical molecules in the air. However, the apple slice can be somewhat protected from the oxidation by lemon juice, which contains antioxidants, especially vitamin C.

You also need to know that there are three very active enzymes called Nitric Oxide Synthases (NOS), which are necessary for your body to manufacture NO. Certain conditions or disorders in the body lead to the production of molecules that inhibit the three NOS enzymes needed to manufacture NO. It's important to know this about NOS, because evidence suggests that antioxidants can boost NO production by directly supporting the production of NOS enzymes.

In a nutshell, scientifically balanced nutritional supplements can both boost production and preserve NO in the body You'll learn more about nutritional supplements later on; first, it's important for you to understand why we prescribe *The Wellness Solution*—and who needs it.

Who Needs The Wellness Solution?

Cardiovascular disease kills more Americans than any other disease does. Therefore, it is crucial to understand how *The Wellness Solution* can help reduce your risk of having a heart attack or stroke. Indeed, people with chronic degenerative diseases anywhere in the body are good candidates for *The Wellness Solution*.

The definition of a risk factor, as used in this book, is something or some action that makes people more likely to have a particular medical problem. Let's consider that notion more carefully. Several relatively recent articles in the *Journal of the American Medical Association* (2003) debunk the long-held myth that only 50 percent of patients with severe heart disease have known risk factors. Instead, the surprising new studies show that about 90 percent of patients with heart disease have one or more of the following risk factors:

> ➢ Obesity
> ➢ Sedentary Lifestyle (Not Enough Exercise)
> ➢ Diabetes Mellitus
> ➢ High Cholesterol or Abnormal Lipids (Fats)
> ➢ High Blood Pressure
> ➢ Smoking

The following risk factors also increase the chance of a heart attack or stroke:

> ➢ Angina or Previous Heart Attack
> ➢ Chronic Stress
> ➢ Age Older than 50 Years
> ➢ Family History of Heart Disease

We definitely prescribe *The Wellness Solution* for anyone with one or more of the above risk factors. NO is ubiquitous in our bodies; there is much more NO than oxygen in us, so it should come as no surprise that this signaling molecule can have so many positive effects—not only for those who are at risk for cardiovascular disease, but for the entire spectrum of chronic degenerative diseases.

A New Psychological Principle

New medical research indicates that our mind-sets and the steps we are willing to take to change our lives for the better can help boost production of NO in the endothelium as well as in the nerve cells of our brain. This means the psychological benefits of NO can be as important as its physical benefits.

The connection between the brain and body occurs when NO is produced in the nerve cells of the brain, specifically the thinking front part, called the cerebrum. Being happy, thinking positive thoughts, and managing stress appear to boost NO production. As a matter of fact, laughing and even humming to yourself have been shown to boost NO production.

NO gas molecules can instantaneously pass right through countless billions of cell membranes that separate the "thinking" cerebrum from the back part of the brain, where the "non-thinking" medulla regulates the body's autonomic nervous system, which controls your heart rate, blood pressure, breathing, stress hormone levels, and virtually everything that happens automatically in the body. Thus, NO sends its signals throughout the brain to the entire body, encouraging homeostasis or entropy.

NO is called a neurotransmitter when it functions in the brain or nerve cells, because it allows the cells to communicate . . . literally to talk with one another. When researchers first explored the roles of NO, the brain was the least expected organ in which to find this gas. Nevertheless, NO is found throughout the entire brain, suggesting its involvement in virtually every brain function as a signaling molecule, spreading messages throughout the brain and body.

That's not all. Dr. Salvador Moncada, a respected British NO researcher, suggests that NO may even be the basis of memory! This idea is based on the discovery that when brain cells are strongly stimulated by NO signals sent from other cells, they produce and send back even more NO molecules to tell the sender cells that their message has been received. Not only that, NO seems to somehow program the sender cells to send even stronger signals the next time. Thus, NO may explain memory formation as well as memory reinforcement.

Reinforcing memory is especially important when people are ready to fall off the wagon regarding their commitments to live healthier lives, for example, by exercising regularly or not smoking or avoiding junk food. We've all experienced how easy it is to talk ourselves into breaking our healthy promises to ourselves by just thinking, *This promise is becoming much too difficult to keep.* Fortunately, NO seems to signal our brain cells to quickly remember why we made the healthy commitment in the first place! In addition, NO may transmit increasingly stronger signals to remind the brain cells about what's important.

To sum up the research, attitude and commitment are real answers to boosting NO in the body, including the brain. A happy, positive attitude in the thinking part of the brain can trigger healthy responses in the autonomic nervous system that decrease stress in the entire body. This can lead to a happier, less stressed, and more positive you.

Rather than giving in to destructive thinking that tells you that enjoying healthy nutrition, managing weight, drinking enough water, taking scientifically balanced nutritional supplements, getting regular exercise, refraining from smoking, and managing stress, including being a good person, are habits that are too difficult to continue, you can let NO help program your thinking brain cells to become even *more* committed to healthy lifestyle changes. What a great bonus when times get tough! The bottom line is that NO is a major key to good health, and the happier and more positive you are, the more NO you will produce.

A New Spiritual Principle

Again, people with more NO in their body are generally healthier than people with less NO. Therefore, it's appropriate to consider all means, natural and medical, to keep your endothelium healthy, boosting NO in your body. But we should ask ourselves: *What is it that stops us from doing what we obviously know we need to do to stay healthy or get well?* We should also ask ourselves: *Why are countless millions of Americans joining the legions of the "worried well" and the "walking wounded"?* We should also wonder why we are becoming a nation of hypochondriacs who are seeking magic pills for everything bothersome. Perhaps part of the answer may be a lack of love for ourselves and others—a feeling of emptiness or spiritual isolation. Being *ill* may sometimes be synonymous with "I Lack Love" (I-L-L), because if we don't value ourselves, we're not very likely to take the necessary steps to improve our health.

Our health is largely determined by personal responsibility, self-value, and reverence for life. That's why being a good person and trying not to do anything wrong are such important ingredients of *The Wellness Solution*.

It's been said that there are no atheists in foxholes, so perhaps the lesson here for all of us is to develop a genuine reverence for life that brings forth the feeling that we are part of something much greater than ourselves . . . a feeling that makes us feel worthy of this life, being alive, and feeling well.

Jerome Groopman, M.D., a respected professor of medicine at the Harvard Medical School, wrote an essay in the *New England Journal of Medicine* about his patient Anna, who was on the cancer ward. Anna asked him to pray to God with her. The doctor considered the fact that none of his training in medical school or medical practice had taught him how to reply to Anna. He began wondering whether doctors should regularly consider religion in the lives of their patients and in their own lives. Mostly he wondered whether there was any place for God at the bedside of the patient during hospital rounds. Facing Anna, he searched for a response and reminded himself that as a physician, whatever he says or does must be for the benefit of his patients. He also contemplated the fact that although the issue of prayer and healing has captured the public's imagination, the published research has been inconclusive. Unsure of which words were appropriate, he asked Anna, "What is the prayer that you want?" "Pray to God to give my doctors wisdom," Anna replied. To that, the doctor silently echoed, "Amen." *So do we.*

The Breakout Principle

Dr. Herbert Benson, also a professor of medicine at the Harvard Medical School, coined a term for the creative breakthrough felt by artists, athletes, students, writers, poets, musicians, and virtually everyone at some time in their lives. He calls the feeling the "Breakout Principle." Research shows the feeling is associated with an increase of NO in the blood and brain. Isn't that just amazing? An increase in NO is also associated with the wonderful feeling of radical amazement that we sometimes experience when we find ourselves taking time to contemplate being part of something larger than us and sacred.

If having a spiritual epiphany is associated with an increase in NO, could it be possible that the vision of a white light at the end of a tunnel, seen by many people while having a near-death experience, is a reflection of the ultimate detonation of NO in the body, signaling life rather than death? Finally, since NO signals both life and death, would it be reasonable to speculate that a higher power helps heal the human body through NO . . . the Spark of Life?

Turning Over a New Leaf

Now that you have learned how important it is to keep your NO levels high, we want to provide a response to a powerful challenge by Dr. Alexander Leaf, who is one of Harvard's most distinguished professors of medicine—and our own medical mentor. Fifteen years ago, Dr. Leaf wrote an essay in the *New England Journal of Medicine* called "The Prevention of Coronary Artery Disease; A Medical Imperative."

Dr. Leaf wrote, "Members of the public need to accept more responsibility for their own health through the choices they make and the lifestyles they pursue. They need to be disabused of the fantasies that they can indulge in whatever lifestyle they wish and that medicine will provide a pill or operation to erase the adverse effects of a lifetime of self-abuse. Achieving cultural change is not easy, but the public is seeking sound advice, so physicians should be in the vanguard."

Dr. Leaf continued, "We realize that risk factors are only crude, sometimes distant, markers of disease, yet we anticipate new and powerful insight into the prevention of disease . . . and physicians are in an optimal position to provide new understanding that will create simpler, more available, more effective preventive measures."

Suddenly, the risk factors Dr. Leaf refers to are no longer "only crude, sometimes distant, markers of disease," because now we know that 90 percent of patients with severe heart disease have identifiable risk factors. As physicians, we also know our principal responsibility is improving our patients' chances for healthy lives. Now, working hand in hand with a uniquely experienced publisher, we humbly accept Dr. Leaf's challenge "to provide new understanding that will create simpler, more available, more effective preventive measures." *This is The Wellness Solution.*

Please read on, and remember that health is your most precious asset.

PART TWO

VITAMINS AND MINERALS: SUSTAINING LIFE

Generalized Hypovitaminosis

We have identified a new disease condition that we believe is a major contributing cause of the rising tide of chronic degenerative diseases in the modern world.

We call this abnormal condition Generalized Hypovitaminosis. It's an aspect of the Taub-Murad-Oliphant Syndrome that we'll tell you more about in the last part of the book. The miracle is the fact that we already have an effective prevention and treatment plan to share with you!

In the United States, we are seeing a startling increase in a long list of such diseases. The list includes Alzheimer's disease; arthritis; autoimmune diseases; blindness from age-related macular degeneration; cataracts; cancer; chronic liver, lung, and kidney diseases; diabetes; osteoporosis; and especially cardiovascular diseases, including atherosclerosis, hypertension, strokes, and heart attacks. Quite a list! As life expectancy continues to increase, as it undoubtedly will, the incidence of these and other degenerative disorders will as well.

We are confident that raising public awareness of Generalized Hypovitaminosis can help to stem this troubling tide by helping hundreds of millions of people who are needlessly suffering with these conditions to avoid the onset of these degenerative diseases and to improve their symptoms.

Generalized Hypovitaminosis sounds pretty complicated. It isn't. Let's break it down and make the definition very clear. It's actually derived from Greek and Latin: *Hypo* means "less than normal," or insufficient. *Vita* means "life." *Amine* refers to nitrogen compounds. *Osis* means "an abnormal condition, disease, or syndrome." Clearly put: This is a disorder caused by having insufficient amounts of vitamins to support Nitric Oxide levels and a healthy life.

Let's look at another example to further clarify Generalized Hypovitaminosis: People with normal levels of NO in their bodies are generally healthier than people with low levels of NO in their bodies. The amount of vitamins that most people consume daily is sufficient to prevent classic vitamin deficiency diseases, such as scurvy, beriberi, pernicious anemia, rickets, and pellagra. But the damage to your body that's caused by increased amounts of free radicals requires increased amounts of vitamins, especially antioxidants. Therefore, when your daily intake of vitamins is insufficient to overcome that damage, the levels of NO in your body decrease, which contributes to the development of chronic degenerative diseases. This is Generalized Hypovitaminosis.

It's really simple to understand. Look at it this way: When your immune system starts to break down, you are susceptible to colds and more serious ailments and sicknesses. If your body is lacking the vitamins and minerals it needs to sustain life, then your immune system starts to weaken and you become vulnerable. The same thing can occur with other bodily systems, not just your immune system. Thus, Generalized Hypovitaminosis can lead to a general systems breakdown that causes chronic degenerative disease in the cardiovascular system, nervous system, hormonal system, gastrointestinal system, genital-urinary system, the bones, and joints. It really is that simple.

Speaking of simple, Generalized Hypovitaminosis, which is a part of the Taub-Murad-Oliphant (TMO) Syndrome, will be called GH in this book from this point on.

Before we go any further, however, let's discuss why we recommend

that you take a well-balanced, scientifically current, and medically responsible vitamin and mineral nutritional system formula.

Our bodies cannot survive without vitamins and minerals, but did
you know that, for the most part, your body doesn't manufacture its own
vitamins and minerals? You only get these essential nutrients from the
foods you eat or the nutritional supplements you ingest. However, even
if you eat very well, it's highly unlikely that you will get the amount of
vitamins and minerals that medical research now shows can reduce your
risk of many major diseases.

The following is a factual short story that we think is interesting, because it illustrates just how current our knowledge of vitamins and minerals really is. In the 18th century, Great Britain's famous explorer
Captain James Cooke observed that sailors suffering with scurvy improved after eating sauerkraut soaked in lemon juice (vitamin C). But it
wasn't until the 19th century that vitamins and minerals were first discovered. Finally, the classic vitamin deficiency diseases weren't even
identified until the 20th century. Then they were given exotic names like
scurvy, beriberi, pellagra, rickets, and pernicious anemia. What resulted
from all the discoveries was the worldwide prevention and treatment of
many serious diseases. This has had a profound impact on hundreds of
millions, maybe even billions, of people, especially those living in countries where chronic malnutrition is prevalent. Amazingly enough, the
prevention and treatment strategies consisted simply of eating more
healthfully and using supplemental vitamins and minerals.

It's also amazing that by some strange twist of fate, and maybe some
politics to boot, the following U.S. government-mandated statement persists, in spite of very solid evidence to the contrary: "Vitamins and minerals are not intended to treat, cure, or prevent any disease."

Something is seriously wrong! This statement is not acceptable in the
21st century, and we look at it as misleading information from the past that
needs some serious updating. For example, iodine deficiency results in goiter
(enlarged thyroid) and hypothyroidism in some inland countries where
seafood is not part of the diet. Iodine supplementation prevents this disorder.

The situation reminds us of a time, not so long ago, when polio began disappearing as a result of Dr. Jonas Salk's famous "dead-virus vaccine"—a world-shaking medical solution that initially caused influential medical scientists and governmental health departments to essentially declare, *Hogwash! It couldn't possibly be effective.* The prevailing medical wisdom discounted the idea that a dead-virus vaccine could inoculate people against getting a disease caused by a live virus. With the help of President Franklin D. Roosevelt and the nonprofit March of Dimes crusade, Dr. Salk's vaccine prevailed . . . and probably saved a whole generation of young people from contracting polio.

We are confident that the updated information that will follow in this part of the book will enlighten you and withstand the test of time. We want to make it clear that it is not our intention to make disease-related claims that fall outside of the U.S. government's regulatory protocols for nutritional supplements. Indeed, our sole intention is to identify the characteristics of a new disease condition, GH, which by its definition may be prevented or treated with the proper use of vitamins and minerals, under a comprehensive umbrella of good medical care and a healthy lifestyle.

However, it's imperative that GH is taken very seriously, which requires new guidelines on prevention and treatment with the proper use of vitamins and minerals. You are about to read, in Part Four of this book, how *The Wellness Solution* deals with reducing the risk of chronic degenerative diseases by fostering your internal healing force—homeostasis—while slowing down the force of entropy that causes everything in the body to eventually fall apart. As a matter of fact, you are about to step outside the traditional disease treatment model of medicine and step into the world of modern preventive medicine and wellness, not illness.

How Common Is Generalized Hypovitaminosis?

GH is widespread throughout the world, but it's especially prevalent in the United States. Ironically, it is a malnutrition disorder that is found mostly in the more "civilized" countries with the most pollution, smog, acid rain, radiation, and stress. It's hard to believe that Americans, living in a culture of supersized meals, could be suffering with a malnutrition disorder, but that's exactly what happens when we make food choices that result in our getting more than a third of our daily calories from unwholesome and unhealthful sources—which they are when they come from fast foods, junk foods, refined sugars, and dangerous fats. These factors contribute to this malnutrition disorder and play a part in breaking down the various systems in our bodies, thus leading to chronic degenerative diseases.

Let us provide a clearly documented example of how dietary changes, diminished exercise, and more sedentary behavior have markedly changed the presence of a serious and common disease, diabetes mellitus. The Pima Indians, for centuries, were a society who actively hunted and raised crops and grains in southwestern areas of North America. They were healthy with only rare cases of diabetes. When they were placed on the reservations, their hunting and agricultural activities diminished. Their diet changed from fruits and grains to more carbohydrates, additional fat-enriched meats, and increased alcohol consumption. Exercise decreased dramatically. Today, the prevalence of diabetes can be as great as 70 percent in some Pima families.

In the United States, the medical concept of hypovitaminosis D surfaced in 2001 with the publication of a very surprising study demonstrating that although rickets—the classic vitamin D deficiency disease—has virtually disappeared, there is new evidence of widespread vitamin D deficiency in old and sick people, because of their limited exposure to sunshine as well as their poor vitamin D intake from food. In a major New England hospital, 57 percent of the elderly patients in the medical wards were found to have significantly low levels of vitamin D in their blood . . . again, the beginning of potential medical problems, including chronic degenerative diseases.

As we've said before, *it is highly unlikely that we will get the vitamins and minerals science now shows us that we need from just the foods we eat.*

Let's continue. Again, even though we may be malnourished, it doesn't always mean that we will have one of the classic vitamin deficiency diseases like beriberi (vitamin B-6), scurvy (vitamin C), pernicious anemia (vitamin B-12), pellagra (vitamin B-6), or rickets (vitamin D), but the situation could lead to GH and then to chronic degenerative diseases.

Another dramatic example was how startled medical scientists were when they discovered that the rate of devastating neural tube birth defects, such as spina bifida, plunged by 80 percent once pregnant women without any signs of classic folic acid deficiency began supplementing their usual diet with just tiny amounts of folic acid. Could this have been a fluke? No, because just a few years later, a dramatic 42 percent reduction in the risk of heart disease was also reported in people who were taking folic acid and vitamin B-6 supplements—even though they had no signs of folic acid or vitamin B-6 deficiency!

Other studies have shown that vitamin C and vitamin E supplements can reduce the risk of heart disease in people without the classic signs of vitamin deficiencies. Also, solid evidence has emerged to show that vitamin C and folic acid supplements reduce the risk of cancer—again, in people without any signs of vitamin deficiency.

Finally, in a recent dramatic study, supplemental antioxidants (vitamins C and E and beta-carotene) and zinc were given to thousands of people who were at increased risk for age-related macular degeneration (the most common cause of blindness in the United States). The following press release (2001) by the National Institutes of Health speaks volumes about GH:

Antioxidant Vitamins and Zinc Reduce Risk of Vision Loss from Age-Related Macular Degeneration

"High levels of antioxidants and zinc significantly reduce the risk of advanced age-related macular degeneration (AMD) and its associated vision loss. Scientists found that people at high risk of developing advanced stages of AMD, a leading cause of vision loss, lowered their risk by about 25 percent when treated with high dosages of vitamin C, vitamin E, beta-carotene, and zinc. This is an exciting discovery because, for people at high risk of developing AMD, these nutrients are the first effective treatment to slow the progression of the disease."

So you can clearly see how the rising tide of chronic degenerative diseases is associated with GH. What is even more remarkable is the fact that preventing and treating GH is such a simple way to reduce your risk of succumbing to such major diseases!

It is interesting to note that GH has certain parallels with another disease, Kwashiorkor, a malnutrition disorder caused by protein deficiency. Kwashiorkor occurs mostly in poverty-stricken countries and is one of the world's most widespread nutritional problems. Its most prominent features are growth failure, muscle loss, generalized swelling, decreased immunity, and a very large, protuberant abdomen. The earliest symptoms are fatigue, tiredness, and lethargy.

Kwashiorkor and GH are both diseases of malnutrition and reflections of the societies in which people live. Kwashiorkor is rampant in the poorest countries, where people are starving, while GH is the scourge of modern countries, where people get enough nutrients to prevent Kwashiorkor but not enough to prevent the chronic degenerative diseases that result from having excess free radicals constantly bombard their cells, because of the so-called good life they lead.

An "essential" nutrient is one that the body cannot make, and its absence from the diet causes disease or even death. Both Kwashiorkor and GH are caused by inadequate intakes of a wide array of essential nutrients. In Kwashiorkor, the deficiencies involve a cluster of amino acids that the body requires to make proteins (lysine, leucine, isoleucine, methionine, and so on). Similarly, we have accurately identified a cluster of vitamin insufficiencies (D, C, E, B-12, B-6, folic acid, and others) as the basis for the condition we now call GH.

Did you know that in the 20th century, cardiovascular disease changed from being a relatively inconsequential disease to a leading cause of disease and death in developed countries? At the beginning of the 20th century, cardiovascular disease accounted for less than 10 percent of all deaths. At the beginning of the 21st century, it accounts for nearly one-half of all deaths in the developed world!

It is indeed ironic that the serious deficiency diseases that were once the common, dreaded hallmarks of vitamin and mineral deficiency have all but disappeared, except in famine-stricken regions of the world. Instead, the endothelial linings of the blood vessels of people in the wealthiest countries in the world are showing signs of disease. People are not producing NO well enough to relax their blood vessel walls and boost homeostasis. That is, in a large part, because they are not getting enough vitamins and minerals from the foods they eat. This is true especially when diets consist of processed junk food—with french fries considered a major source of vegetables. That's outrageous!

Let's continue along our path to a healthier you. People who are most susceptible to GH are those with one or more of the risk factors for cardiovascular disease that we identify in Parts One and Four of this book. Also highly susceptible are people with long-standing illnesses, especially cancer or conditions associated with weight loss or poor nutrition. Pregnancy, breast-feeding, the use of multiple prescription drugs, the frequent use of antacids, and alcoholism all increase the chances of vitamin deficiency. Undoubtedly, severe psychological stress—such as a divorce, the loss of a loved one, the loss of a job—also increases susceptibility to GH.

Let's recap: GH is a malnutrition disorder caused by vitamin intakes that are insufficient to combat the oxidative stress of modern times and the general damage caused by free-radical molecules. This causes endothelial damage, inflamed arteries, and decreased levels of NO throughout the entire body. In ample quantity, NO supports homeostasis. On the other hand, an insufficient quantity of NO encourages entropy. We've already discussed homeostasis and entropy, but we want to discuss the subject in more depth because your understanding of these forces, which are responsible for your life, is crucial to your successful compliance with *The Wellness Solution*.

Medical scientists have discovered that our cells have a built-in mechanism to destroy themselves . . . literally to commit suicide. The phenomenon is called apoptosis (*ay-pop-TOE-sis*). It's a part of the force called entropy, which causes everything to eventually fall apart.

To repeat, in ample quantity, NO supports homeostasis. An insufficient quantity of NO encourages entropy by initiating apoptosis, our cells' built-in program to destroy their cells. In a sense, apoptosis is the handmaiden of entropy. This is important for you to understand, because each of your cells is regulated by a biological clock in your DNA. Some people's DNA leads to diabetes, hypertension, and heart disease; other people's DNA leads to chronic liver, lung, or kidney disease. In any case, as you age, especially after your reproductive years, entropy normally begins overtaking homeostasis. Thus, nature phases out old life for new life. The balance between the forces of homeostasis and entropy is the life story of every creature. It determines how healthy and long we will live.

Decreased NO production sends a signal for apoptosis to start so entropy begins taking over. Medical science merely puts *labels* on the consequences of apoptosis: heart attack (myocardial infarction), hypertension, stroke, diabetes mellitus, cancer, arthritis, osteoporosis, age-related macular degeneration, nephritis, lupus erythematosus, Alzheimer's syndrome, Parkinson's disease, and so on. Not a very pretty list.

What Are Signs of Generalized Hypovitaminosis?

As we have noted, GH is a major contributing cause of common chronic degenerative diseases. Newly emerging studies suggest it may also be associated with chronic infections such as herpes and tuberculosis. We also suspect that various poorly understood diseases, such as fibromyalgia and chronic fatigue syndrome, may be involved.

The signs and symptoms of GH may include fatigue, lethargy, weakness, forgetfulness, moodiness, and anxiety. Often there is a sense of "something missing or wrong" in the quality of life—there's *less energy, zest, and vitality.* Other symptoms can include poor attention span, cravings for sweets, drug and alcohol abuse, and compulsive behavior. Some people may even notice their hair falling out and their nails growing more slowly than normal.

There are no well-accepted, established criteria for the diagnosis of this new syndrome. It's a complex disorder and an emerging clinical challenge, so we look forward to seeing help from many medical experts providing specific guidelines in the future.

In the meantime, since NO is so fundamentally important in regulating biological processes and is relatively difficult to measure at specific sites in the body, GH is primarily a diagnosis of inclusion. This means that GH is so widespread that it should be considered as a contributing cause of chronic degenerative diseases affecting all parts of the body.

Obviously, GH should be especially suspected with any of the high-risk factors for coronary artery disease that have been previously listed. GH usually develops slowly, but it can develop rapidly during periods of increased susceptibility, such as pregnancy, breast-feeding, use of multiple medications, drug and alcohol abuse, smoking, severe stress, and relentless fear and worry. GH can also develop rapidly during all types of chronic illnesses or infections and can worsen the conditions so much that they become life threatening.

We are not in any way trying to scare you. Really, we only want to make you better informed about what you can do to help yourself be a healthier you!

Let's continue. Specific blood tests may be helpful. For example, blood tests may reveal elevated levels of homocysteine, C-reactive protein, triglycerides, cholesterol, and LDL. On the other hand, levels of hemoglobin, HDL, folate, and vitamin B-12 are commonly lower.

Positive blood tests for autoimmune conditions may be useful, including serum complement, immune globulins, rheumatoid factor, and lupus factor. Urine testing may show abnormal albumin. It may sound a bit overwhelming to you, but your personal doctor will fully understand this information if you bring it to his or her attention.

We recommend that you have thorough physical examinations periodically, including complete histories, especially regarding food intake and lifestyle patterns. However, if the index of suspicion for GH is high—even if it's just based on your plain old common sense—then little time should be lost before starting *The Wellness Solution*, because it is so safe, beneficial, and inexpensive. By the way, Personal Evaluation (Part Five) is not a bad way to start!

How Is Generalized Hypovitaminosis Prevented and Treated?

The proper management of GH includes ongoing medical care and a healthy lifestyle regimen. For instance, patients with hypertension need adequate blood pressure control; patients with diabetes require tight control of blood glucose; patients who are at increased risk for cardiovascular disease should discuss the use of aspirin and cholesterol-lowering drugs (statins) with their physicians.

Aspirin helps prevent blood clots that form as a result of endothelial dysfunction and then cause heart attacks and strokes. Statins improve endothelial health because high cholesterol causes more free radicals, which harm the endothelium. Statins also stimulate Nitric Oxide Synthase (NOS) enzymes that lead to increased production of NO. Remember, sufficient NO, among other effects, causes the blood vessels to relax and widen, thereby improving blood flow to the heart and all over the body.

There Are No Magic Pills

In any case, a sound nutritional supplement system can provide a dietary safety net, but it does not even come close to making up for unhealthful eating habits. In other words, supplements cannot replace the immeasurable benefits of eating fresh fruits, vegetables, and whole grains.

As we will say many times in this book, *even if you eat very well, it is highly unlikely that you will get enough of the vitamins and minerals that science now shows you need to prevent or treat GH and its consequences.* However, eating well is critical to your well-being, and a sound nutritional supplement system should complement your food intake, not replace it!

As we've said before, our trillions of cells constantly contend with renegade, electron-stealing free radicals that oxidize and cause damage to our DNA, to the inside of our blood vessel walls, to the proteins in our eyes and to virtually everywhere else in the body. Obviously, preventing and treating GH requires more than just a nutritional supplement formula. It also requires a solid commitment from you to accept personal responsibility for helping to determine your own health destiny through *The Wellness Solution*.

If you have a chronic degenerative disease that has not progressed too far, the prognosis can usually be improved. However, even if a disease is in the advanced stages, we are still confident that your knowledge and proper actions can lead to an increased sense of well-being that's better than you could have ever imagined. By taking proper action, you should be able to sense a positive difference in two weeks and feel a definite difference in a month. So ask yourself if you're willing to do what it takes. If you are ready to feel better and be healthier, then let's proceed!

Delivering Life

NO signaling is one of the most rapidly growing areas in medical research, because it regulates a vast array of biological processes needed for life. Dr. Murad's discovery has expanded the treatment options for doctors entrusted with patient care as much as the discovery of oxygen did. It's a wonderful addition to what doctors call their therapeutic armamentarium. When Dr. Murad discovered that nitroglycerin works by releasing NO molecules, he opened the door to one of the most exciting opportunities in the history of modern medicine: **sustaining life . . . through the delivery of NO, to open the doors that will allow the free flow of oxygen to our cells!**

The oxygen molecule supports life by hitching onto the hemoglobin molecules in the blood and then nourishing the cells at the end of our blood vessels—the tiny capillaries. The NO molecule helps to sustain life by relaxing and opening those blood vessels to get oxygen to our cells. Every 60 seconds, our blood vessels distribute five quarts of blood—carrying oxygen from our lungs—to our cells. That's about 600,000 gallons a year . . . an ocean of life.

But the key is that our blood vessels must be relaxed and open. When they are not relaxed, then our blood flow is severely diminished and the arteries become inflamed, especially when the tiny capillaries are affected. This is basically what occurs with GH and decreased levels of NO.

A good example of the consequences of decreased NO is the recent discovery that endothelial dysfunction appears to be a major cause of adult-onset diabetes. It's been demonstrated that capillary narrowing due to decreased NO levels leads to insulin resistance in the body's cells . . . hence, adult-onset diabetes.

Remember, Dr. Murad discovered that nitroglycerin works by releasing puffs of NO molecules, which cause the smooth muscles in the walls of the coronary arteries to relax. It is the same with the rest of the body. Before this discovery, NO was thought to be a toxic gas that existed only outside the body—mostly in car exhaust fumes and smoke from factory chimneys due to the combustion of fossil fuels. Now we know there are more Nitric Oxide molecules in the body than oxygen molecules!

NO acts as the signaling molecule for the body by carrying its chemical messages within cells and between cells. Dr. Murad discovered that NO gas activates an enzyme that makes a compound called cyclic GMP, which relaxes the delicate smooth muscle cells in blood vessel walls to keep them open. Viagra works by enhancing the action of cyclic GMP by preventing its inactivation, thereby improving blood flow in the arteries of the penis. The prevention and treatment of GH is also based on cyclic GMP and on boosting NO levels to improve the blood flow in all of the arteries throughout the body—whether male or female—to sustain life.

NO is ubiquitous. NO is in our bloodstreams and inside our cells. NO is in our brains and nerves. NO helps relax the smooth muscles of our airways so we can breathe. NO relaxes the smooth muscle of our intestines so we digest our food. NO is crucial for our memory and probably our feelings. NO helps our kidneys to function, supports our eyesight, combats infection, and even acts as a master hormone in our bodies. There are no other molecules in nature that can serve such diverse roles as NO!

You could choose a place almost anywhere in the human body and NO would be there. Besides Viagra, there are countless other valuable nuggets to be discovered in the vast gold mine of NO biology. That's what makes the study of GH so incredibly interesting.

In our wellness medical practice, which we describe more fully later on in this book, another healing dimension is added: *fostering homeostasis by regulating apoptosis and slowing down entropy.* This healing dimension requires a common belief or hope—shared by both patients and their doctors—that in addition to good medicine, your health is largely determined by personal responsibility, self-value, and reverence for life.

Simply put, this means your health largely depends on what you're willing to do for yourself. The great beauty of *The Wellness Solution* is that it works by stimulating our own internal healing resources. An easy way to start the process is by taking a scientifically well-balanced nutritional system formula over the long term, in conjunction with *The Wellness Solution.*

Why Should Supplement Buyers Be Very Careful?

The nutritional industry is so poorly regulated that it's fraught with non-sense and various fads of the month, often generating sales for products that are useless and potentially harmful. A good example is the recent coral calcium craze that generated hundreds of millions of dollars in revenues through TV infomercials touting its benefits for virtually all our ills. Finally, the Federal Trade Commission stepped in to ban further sales because of the worthless claims. Weight-loss products are also memorable examples of the amount of money that people pay for products that do not work, such as garcinia cambogia, chromium picolinate, vanadium, starch blockers, fat burners, and lately the "growth-hormone activators," all unproven and generally worthless. Of course, what's worse than bilking the public, especially the elderly, of money, is the loss of countless lives from the unregulated use of ephedrine supplements for weight loss and energy.

Vitamin A is another example of potential harm. It's disturbing to note that the vitamin supplement industry has, for the most part, paid little attention to the surprising scientific findings published in the *New England Journal of Medicine* in 2002. A study following 2,300 men in Sweden taking vitamin A supplements for over 30 years demonstrated that vitamin A may weaken bones and increase the risk of fractures. The findings confirmed yet another study by Harvard Medical School researchers following over 80,000 female nurses for over 20 years. They discovered that higher intakes of Vitamin A among the nurses were associated with more broken hips and weak bones.

The studies raised a serious concern about the safety of taking vitamin A supplements over the long term. It's a concern clearly voiced in the accompanying editorial in the *New England Journal of Medicine:* "The study suggests that vitamin A supplementation and fortification of food with vitamin A may be harmful in Western countries, where life expectancy is high and the prevalence of osteoporosis is increasing. . . .

One may conclude from such data that supplements containing vitamin A should not be routinely taken by men or women."

Therefore, adults should not take vitamin A supplements unless they have specific medical reasons for doing so, especially since it's so easily supplied in our daily diet by green leafy vegetables, yellow vegetables, fruits, fish, eggs, and fortified cereals. Once vitamin A is eliminated, then beta-carotene can easily take its place, because your body converts it to a safe form of vitamin A that does not weaken bones over the long term.

In our opinion, the nutritional supplement industry needs to be more proactive by taking proper steps that protect the public against potential negative side effects of supplements. Then for the industry, as well as the consumer, the positive effects of supplements can be a major benefit to society in the face of astronomical medical expenses and a health care system that is no longer working primarily to protect the interests of patients.

The quality of evidence that supports the prevention and treatment of GH syndrome is outstanding, not only in terms of the published scientific literature, but also from the clinical experience emerging from over 100,000 individuals who have been taking Dr. Taub's vitamin and mineral nutritional system for years. One consistent finding stands out in both published and strictly clinical research: *Taking a daily well-balanced, comprehensive nutritional system as part of a healthy lifestyle strategy is the key to maintaining optimal health and wellness.*

Nature's Simple Genius

We have formulated guidelines for a sensible nutritional system formula to help prevent and treat GH. We want you to take the formula every day, virtually forever, to promote endothelial health and boost the level of NO in your body, while reducing your risk of getting many diseases. We believe that taking this formula—along with following *The Wellness Solution*—is one of the most effective things that you can do to help determine your own health destiny.

We've applied the same level of scientific vigilance that we normally use for prescription drugs before recommending our nutritional system formula to you, and we feel it's important for you to know that we have used the following guidelines:

- First, do no harm. . . . *Primum non nocere.*
- Always understand an ingredient's molecular basis for action.
- Avoid ingredients without compelling science and evidence for effectiveness.
- Use the most effective yet safest dosages of the ingredients.

The traditional medical model of treatment is based on the scientific study of disease and its causes, consequences, and treatment. The goal of drugs is to treat diseases by modifying biological pathways, sometimes in ways that, unfortunately, cause undesirable side effects. On the other hand, the goal of a nutritional system is to stimulate optimal health and wellness through a more gentle and natural approach.

Therefore, we've gone beyond looking at supplements through the traditional medical model, because it doesn't come close to explaining the beneficial effects we've noted during our 90 combined years of medical practice, teaching, and research. Nor does the medical model explain the lessons learned by Dr. Taub while addressing the vitamin and mineral needs of a television-based Wellness Practice that reaches over 90 million homes. In other words, our personal and professional experience in the real world differs from the following medical cliché taught to doctors for the last hundred years in medical school pharmacology courses: "Patients who take supplemental vitamins and minerals are just enriching their urine."

We welcomed the conclusion of a review in the prestigious *Journal of the American Medical Association* (JAMA), published in 2002, which concluded that *all adults should be taking a daily multivitamin and mineral supplement.*

As you already know, our bodies do not manufacture vitamins and minerals. Therefore, we must get them through the foods or the supplements we take. That's the reason why nutritional supplements, especially antioxidants, are so important. But remember, *even if you eat very well, it's highly unlikely that you would get the optimal amount of vitamins and minerals that science now shows us is needed to prevent or treat GH.* Nevertheless, please read the following very carefully: **A poor diet supplemented with the very best nutritional supplement system is still a poor diet.**

More About Free Radicals and Antioxidants

Let's start piecing together what we have so far, especially as it relates to cardiovascular disease and other chronic degenerative diseases. The high-risk factors listed in Part One of this book lead directly to the increased production of free radicals. These are unbalanced, highly unstable oxygen molecules that are missing an electron. They cause a wide swath of destruction throughout the entire body by snatching electrons away from perfectly balanced, stable molecules that make up our healthy cells, tissues, and organs. This chemical process is called oxidation, which is the molecular basis of many chronic degenerative diseases. Oxidation is the scientific term for rust. Oxidative stress is the scientific term for the general damage that occurs to your body from free radicals. GH is the result of insufficient vitamin intakes to control oxidative stress. Interesting!

Wellness is more than just the absence of disease. Therefore, wise physicians realize that the natural healing resources of their patients must be combined with the best that medicine has to offer. The nutritional system formula we've formulated can help you stimulate your own internal healing forces to help your body be as strong as possible, helping you fight against the external influences that attack your body every day. This means fostering homeostasis and regulating entropy by increasing NO levels in the body to combat the oxidative stress being caused by free radicals.

Antioxidant vitamins and minerals help protect our bodies against the harmful effects of free-radical damage by inhibiting the formation of free radicals as well as blocking the damage they cause. Although antioxidants help prevent or repair oxidative damage, once the amount of rust that you accumulate exceeds your body's ability to repair it, then chronic degenerative diseases tend to occur.

Remember, every cell in the human body is constantly exposed to free radicals that are normally generated by our daily metabolism, natural aging process, and the fact that we breathe and require oxygen. Problems occur only when there are too many of these renegade electron stealers! A good example is oxidized LDL (low-density lipoproteins), which is the "bad" cholesterol that is primarily responsible for atherosclerosis and inflammation in our arteries. LDL is a mixture of fat, protein . . . and rust!

We've discussed how high-risk factors increase free radicals that inactivate NO. The risk factors can also lead to a decrease in NO by stimulating production of specific molecules that inhibit Nitric Oxide Synthases (NOS). These enzymes are responsible for producing NO. So the bottom line is that ingesting more antioxidants, from food and from nutritional supplements, helps overcome NOS inhibition to increase NO production, helps prevent NO inactivation, and helps restore endothelial health. It should be abundantly clear by now that antioxidants decrease the damage done by free radicals and help to boost the production and beneficial effects of NO in our bodies.

An important study published in the *Journal of the American College of Cardiology* reported that the women in the Harvard Nurses' Health Study who took vitamin C supplements over the long term had a 28 percent lower risk of coronary heart disease than the women who did not take vitamin C supplements. Very surprising was this fact: Risk reduction was related only to the supplements the nurses were taking, not to their vitamin C intake from foods! The accompanying editorial suggested that vitamin C lowers cardiovascular risk by maintaining normal endothelial function and increasing NO activity.

The potential benefits of increasing NO in our bodies are far-ranging, because relaxing the blood vessels and keeping them open helps ensure delivery of life-giving oxygen to all of the body's cells and organs. After all, think about this. . . . The human body is such a finely tuned living system that death occurs when we stop breathing oxygen for only five minutes. That's just the loss of about a hundred breaths of oxygen in a system designed for a *billion* breaths over a lifetime! A more gradual loss of oxygen results in inflammation, pain, illness, and disease.

Again, it's very basic: NO helps ensure oxygen delivery, but excess free radicals decrease NO and compromise the delivery of oxygen. You can't see them or feel them, but unfortunately, our modern lifestyles can cause an explosion of free radicals that cause our cells, tissues, and organs to rust away.

The good news is that there is a solution, but we must repeat that the key is still your willingness to take responsibility for your own health destiny. Remember, the body is always seeking balance. It balances homeostasis, our healing force, with the force of entropy, which, as we told you earlier, leads to programmed cell death—apoptosis. Just think: homeostasis versus entropy . . . life and death . . . with each force largely regulated by the presence or absence of NO.

Vitamins and minerals are part of nature's simple genius to help maintain your body's energy balance, but there are no magic pills. There is only good medical science and your willingness to follow *The Wellness Solution*, which consists of healthy nutrition, weight management, adequate amounts of water, regular exercise, not smoking, and stress management, which includes being a good person . . . plus taking a scientifically balanced vitamin and mineral nutritional system formula.

About 100,000 scientific studies on NO have been published since Dr. Murad first described the biological effect of NO, which resulted in his winning the Nobel Prize. Perhaps the even bigger prize—for the ultimate benefit of humankind as well as for the advancement of science—is the fact that Dr. Murad's discovery provides the molecular basis for combining the traditional medical model of treating disease with the wellness medical model of stimulating health and preventing disease. We now know that NO gas diffuses everywhere in the body, creating an invisible mist of chemical sparks signaling health and wellness. Unleashing such power can bring us wonderful benefits. Let's start with the key vitamins that promote endothelial health and nitric oxide production.

Vitamin C

Vitamin C is one of the most proven antioxidants on Planet Earth. We mentioned this example before, but now we'd like you to try this little experiment: Slice an apple in half, and then apply lemon juice to the surface of one half and leave the other half alone. Only the surface of the untreated half will turn brown from oxidation. That's because the vitamin C in lemon is an antioxidant with remarkable ability to reduce the havoc and rust that are caused by the renegade free radicals that steal electrons from other healthy molecules.

In the body, vitamin C helps build healthy bones and teeth, promote wound healing and tissue repair, and much more. It also appears to be somewhat effective in cleaning up damage from cigarette smoke . . . *but we are NOT saying it's OK to smoke if you take vitamin C!*

Vitamin C plays a pivotal role in supporting endothelial health, endothelial function, and NO production. Vitamin C even improves endothelial health when free-radical damage is already present. The beneficial effects of vitamin C actually increase in patients with coronary artery disease. Vitamin C is also especially effective in people who are obese, who smoke, who have an imbalance in their blood sugar, or who need to maintain a healthy blood pressure.

It's worth repeating that the female nurses who took vitamin C supplements over the long term had a 28 percent lower risk of coronary heart disease than the women who did not take vitamin C supplements. In some studies, vitamin C has also increased the effects of nitroglycerin, a NO drug, in patients with angina pectoris.

Not surprisingly, in light of its extraordinary antioxidant power, vitamin C also helps protect against cancer. People with low vitamin C intakes have more cancer of the mouth, larynx, esophagus, breast, lung, stomach, colon, rectum, and cervix than people with higher vitamin C intakes. A large study of people ingesting more than 200 mg of vitamin C per day—again, over the long term—showed a 60 percent reduction in the risk of salivary gland cancer.

There is also strong evidence that vitamin C, along with vitamin E and beta-carotene, reduces the risk of cataracts. Researchers estimate the number of cataract operations could decrease by 50 percent if people ingested adequate amounts of vitamin C. The Harvard Nurses' Health Study demonstrated an 83 percent decrease in the incidence of cataracts among women consuming at least 250 mg of vitamin C for 10 years, as compared to women who were not taking any vitamin C.

No discussion regarding vitamin C would be complete without addressing the common cold. Some studies show that ingesting relatively high doses of vitamin C can reduce the frequency of colds and the duration of the cold symptoms. Other studies contradict these findings. In any case, the authors of this book take 1,000 mg to 1,250 mg of vitamin C daily and double their intake when they feel like they are coming down with a cold.

We recommend a daily intake of 500 to 1,500 mg of vitamin C as part of a scientifically well-balanced vitamin and mineral nutritional system to help reduce the risk of GH.

Folic Acid

Folic acid, another incredible antioxidant, is the B vitamin that stunned and changed the science of nutritional supplements, because it dramatically lowers the risk of birth defects such as spina bifida (an opening in the spine) or anencephaly (absence of the brain). The evidence for this is so strong—it prevents about 80 percent of these birth defects—that all women who are capable of becoming pregnant should take a nutritional supplement with at least 600 mcg of folic acid every day as part of a complete nutritional system.

Folic acid is also important for reducing the risk of cancer. A higher intake reduces the risk of colon and breast cancer, particularly among moderate consumers of alcohol. Men in the "Health Professionals Follow-Up Study" who were taking multivitamins with folic acid for over 10 years demonstrated a 25 percent reduction in the risk of colon cancer.

Even more dramatically, the women in the Harvard Nurses' Health Study who took multivitamins with folic acid for longer than 15 years had a 75 percent reduction in colorectal cancer risk. Higher folic acid intake may also reduce the risk of breast cancer, especially among women who consume alcohol.

Folic acid plays a crucial role in promoting endothelial health and increasing NO production, especially in people with high cholesterol levels. It even helps lessen the endothelial dysfunction that occurs after high-fat meals!

The body requires sufficient levels of folic acid, along with vitamins B-12 and B-6, to help lower homocysteine. High levels of homocysteine may injure the endothelium and cause inflammation and coronary artery disease, regardless of the cholesterol level in the blood. It may even be that depositing fatty matter on the inflamed endothelium is just the body's ill-fated attempt to protect the injury and halt the damage—like a poor bandage.

Americans tend to consume insufficient amounts of B vitamins, leading to high levels of homocysteine, especially among older people. Smoking and heavy coffee drinking also increase homocysteine, but the single most important factor leading to high homocysteine levels appears to be an insufficient intake of folic acid and vitamins B-6 and B-12.

It's remarkable to note that the women in the Harvard Nurses' Health Study who consumed 400 mcg of folic acid and 3 mg of vitamin B-6 a day (for 10 years) decreased their incidence of coronary artery disease and heart attack by over 40 percent.

Vitamin B-12

Vitamin B-12, without question, is a very important vitamin for a healthy heart and healthy blood, nerves, and DNA. In spite of such importance, it's remarkable that about 50 percent of people over the age of 60 in North America and Europe are deficient in vitamin B-12. It's found only in animal products, so deficiency can result from poor food intake, strict vegetarianism, or poor absorption in the stomachs of older individuals who produce less hydrochloric acid. About a third of people over age 50 don't produce enough stomach acid; thus, their B-12 absorption is reduced. Consequently, the National Academy of Sciences recommends that people over the age of 50 take oral vitamin B-12 supplements. Most physicians were taught that B-12 could only be given by injection, but oral B-12 works just fine.

Only a very small amount of this vitamin is needed to do its job.

Vitamin B-6 (Pyridoxine)

Vitamin B-6 is required for over a hundred enzyme reactions, especially for protein and hormone metabolism. It's found in a wide variety of plant and animal products: poultry, fish, meat, legumes, nuts, potatoes, and whole grains. An inadequate dietary intake of vitamin B-6 is relatively common, which, as mentioned above, is undoubtedly a major contributing factor to high levels of homocysteine in the blood.

*We recommend a daily intake of 400 mcg to 800 mcg of folic acid, 200 mcg to 600 mcg of vitamin B-12, and 10 mg to 20 mg of vitamin B-6 in the form of a nutritional supplement to reduce the risk of GH leading to coronary artery disease. But again, there are no magic pills, so your compliance with **The Wellness Solution** is essential.*

Vitamin E

Vitamin E is a powerful antioxidant that improves endothelial function and stimulates NO production by protecting cells from the damaging effects of free radicals. In fact, vitamin E may be the "miracle" antioxidant of our times! For example, the Harvard Nurses' Health Study showed specifically that the intake of vitamin E supplements (at least 100 IU per day for two years or longer) was associated with a 41 percent reduction in the risk of coronary artery disease. The Cambridge Heart Antioxidant Study showed that higher dosages (400 IU to 800 IU per day) of vitamin E supplements were associated with a 77 percent reduction in heart attacks during the two-year study. In both these clinical studies, the vitamin E supplements were taken every day over the long term.

Strong evidence also suggests that vitamin E can reduce your risk of cancer. In a study involving over 400 colon cancer patients and a similar number of healthy people, it was found that taking multivitamins containing 200 IU of vitamin E for 10 years was associated with a 57 percent reduction in the risk of colon cancer.

A study published in the *Annals of Internal Medicine* in 2004 that generated headlines seemed to show that very sick people taking 400 IU or more of vitamin E supplements every day had a slightly higher death rate. Here's the real story: The study combined the findings of 19 older studies that failed to show any harm, much less an increase in deaths. However, by combining the older studies, the numbers indicated a tiny increase in "mortality from all causes." This type of study, which combines a bunch of older studies, is called a meta-analysis. Many epidemiologists do not pay much attention to these types of studies because the statisticians are forced to ignore important nuances and findings in each one of the individual studies.

For example, in this meta-analysis, the actual benefits of vitamin E supplements reported in the very same 19 studies were totally ignored.

Those reported benefits include a reduction in the risk of Alzheimer's disease, heart and blood vessel disease, age-related macular degeneration, and several forms of cancer. The increase in mortality reported in this study was so tiny that it was less than *one-half of one percent.* Furthermore, it represented "mortality from *all* causes," which can include earthquakes, floods, famine, homicides, suicides, and accidents. That's pretty ridiculous!

In any case, the Institute of Medicine, which is a division of the National Academy of Sciences, has made a determination that vitamin E supplements are safe in doses up to 1,500 IU a day.

Supplements are an important means of increasing vitamin E consumption, because most of our foods provide only small amounts of this essential antioxidant. A cup of almonds contains about 20 IU of vitamin E, a cup of hazelnuts has about 30 IU. You would need to ingest over three quarts of olive oil a day to provide 400 IU of vitamin E, which is highly unlikely!

We recommend a daily intake of 200 IU to 400 IU of vitamin E in the alpha-tocopherol form in order to reduce your risk of GH.

Coenzyme Q-10 (CoQ-10)

CoQ-10 is also a very powerful antioxidant found in virtually every cell in the body. It's produced by the body and found in high concentrations in the heart, liver, and kidneys. It plays a vital role in the production of energy in cells, triggering the conversion of nutrients into ATP—a fuel for cells to burn. ATP cannot be stored in high enough quantities to sustain optimal bodily functions for more than a few minutes, so the supply of ATP must be continually renewed, making an ample supply of CoQ-10 mandatory.

CoQ-10 is widely used in Japan, where it has been one of the most commonly used, physician-prescribed remedies for congestive heart failure. (It is not approved for such use in the United States.) Since CoQ-10 recently became available without a prescription in Japan, it has become so popular that a worldwide shortage has occurred, and prices are increasing at a rapid rate.

Coenzyme Q-10 supports heart health by providing optimal nutrition at the cellular level. It helps with certain symptoms of heart disease and helps reduce systolic blood pressure in people with hypertension.

A study published in the *Archives of Neurology* in 2004 demonstrated that statin drugs, which are widely used to lower cholesterol, can seriously inhibit the body's production of CoQ-10. The authors believe that the resultant CoQ-10 deficiency may be the cause of the common adverse side effects of the statin drugs—fatigue, severe muscle pain, and muscle breakdown. The study concludes: "Even brief exposure to atorvastatin (Lipitor) causes a marked decrease in blood CoQ-10 concentration." **We believe that the evidence is strong enough so that most patients who are taking statin drugs to lower their risk of heart attacks and strokes should also be taking a CoQ-10 supplement.**

CAUTION: People with heart disease or high blood pressure should always consult with their personal physicians before following any of our recommendations. Also, people taking a statin drug (Lipitor, Pravacol, Mevacor, Vytorin, Crestor, Zetia, and the like) should consult with their physicians regarding the benefits of CoQ-10.

We recommend a daily intake of between 50 mg and 300 mg of CoQ-10 in the form of a nutritional supplement.

Omega-3 Fatty Acids (Fish Oil)

Omega-3 fatty acids are essential elements of human nutrition; however, the body can't make them. One of the best sources for these fatty acids is oil from the tissues of fish. Fish oil has been shown to improve endothelial function and to increase aarterial relaxation. The nurses followed by Harvard Medical School researchers show that a higher consumption of fish and omega-3 fatty acids leads to a lower risk of coronary artery disease. A study published in *Lancet*, one of the most prestigious British medical journals, followed more than 11,000 Italian patients with recent heart attacks over two years. The patients who took a fish oil omega-3 supplement, as opposed to a placebo, showed a 30 percent decrease in deaths from heart disease and strokes.

The American Heart Association (AHA) has issued a comprehensive report examining the health benefits of omega-3 fatty acids. According to the report:

> Omega-3 fatty acids affect heart health in positive ways. They benefit the heart health of healthy people, people at high risk of cardiovascular disease, and patients with cardiovascular disease.

> Increasing omega-3 fatty acid intake through foods is preferable. However, patients with coronary artery disease may not be able to get enough omega-3 fatty acids (about 1 gram per day) by diet alone. These people may want to talk to their doctor about taking a supplement to reduce their risk of coronary heart disease.

We suggest eating fatty fish (salmon, mackerel, sardines, trout, and halibut) two or three times a week. Anyone who is pregnant or lactating, however, should be wary of eating fish with high mercury content. The fetus or baby could be affected. High-quality, enteric-coated supplements should not smell fishy or leave a fishy aftertaste.

We recommend taking a daily supplement of 500 mg to 1200 mg of fish oil with omega-3 fatty acids.

L-Arginine

CAUTION: L-arginine is an amino acid that is necessary for the body to produce NO. But L-arginine is not included in our list of recommended ingredients for a scientifically balanced vitamin and mineral nutritional system formula because of a report published by the *Journal of the American Medical Association* (2006) that casts doubt on both the safety and usefulness of this supplement.

In the report, investigators from the Johns Hopkins Medical School concluded that the use of L-arginine supplements in patients who had previous heart attacks had no benefit and potentially increased the risk of death. As a result, Health Canada, a government agency, has issued a recall on all products that contain L-arginine and do not have an appropriate warning on the label.

Other reputable investigators are seriously questioning the validity of the Hopkins study. Nevertheless, until additional studies are available, it's important to be conservative and cautious. Therefore, people should not take L-arginine supplements unless they are under the supervision of a physician who is aware of the Hopkins study. It is also important to note that migraine-type headaches, presumably due to the dilation of blood vessels, and herpes flare-ups have been reported.

Under no circumstances should L-arginine supplements be used by patients who have had previous heart attacks unless the Hopkins study is disproven.

A Scientifically Balanced Vitamin and Mineral Nutritional System

The intent of this part of the book was not to describe all the essential vitamins and minerals in detail, but rather to present important facts about some of the key ingredients in supplements that are especially important to help prevent and treat Generalized Hypovitaminosis.

Before presenting our overall guidelines and recommendations, it is important to note that men and women tend to have differing needs for different ingredients at different ages. For instance, iron deficiency anemia is relatively common in premenopausal women in America, so an iron supplement is useful for them. But postmenopausal women (those who are not having their period for any reason), as well as men, should not take an iron supplement because it can predispose them to cardiovascular disease, type 2 diabetes and hemochromatosis, which is a condition associated with increased iron in the blood.

Excess iron can also promote the formation of free radicals and may also obscure an anemia due to peptic ulcers or gastrointestinal cancer. Examples of the need for increased dosages of vitamins as we age include vitamin B-12 and vitamin D. Finally, men require more zinc for prostate health but should take lower amounts of calcium than women for the same reason.

We have taken many factors into consideration before presenting you with the following guidelines and recommendations. Indeed, these are the same guidelines that we use for our own health and well-being, and these are the recommendations that we make to our patients, friends, and family.

Choose products only from reputable manufacturers that do not contain vitamin A and that do feature either the NSF (The Public Health and Safety Company™) or the USP (United States Pharmacopeia) logo on the label. NSF and USP standards guarantee purity, potency, and freshness and the dissolution and disintegration of the product in your body.

The following is a list of our guidelines for your daily nutritional system formula.

GUIDELINES FOR NUTRITIONAL SYSTEM FORMULA

- Beta-carotene   2000–4000 IU

- Vitamin B-1   10–20 mg

- Vitamin B-2   10–20 mg

- Vitamin B-6   10–20 mg

- Vitamin B-12   200–800 mcg (*increase with age*)

- Niacin   20–40 mg

- Pantothenic Acid   20–40 mg

- Folic Acid   400–800 mcg

- Vitamin C   500–1500 mg

- Vitamin D   400–1000 IU (*increase with age*)

- Vitamin E   200–400 IU

- Calcium   500–1500 mg (*increase with age*)

- Selenium   200 mcg

- Magnesium   300–600 mg

- Iron   18 mg (*only menstruating women*)

- Zinc   15–40 mg (*more for men*)

- Chromium   80–100 mcg

- Biotin   20–40 mcg

- Lutein   500–1000 mcg

- Lycopene   500–1000 mcg

- CoQ-10   50–300 mg

- Fish Oil/Omega-3   500–1200 mg

A New Beginning . . . Revisited

Remember, one of the goals of *The Wellness Solution* is to help you boost the levels of NO in your blood in order to maintain healthier blood vessels. A very delicate balance exists in the capability of endothelium to relax the vessels and keep them open to deliver blood and oxygen—and life.

Healthy endothelial cells produce, as well as require, ample amounts of NO, so the balance between homeostasis and entropy can vary from moment to moment. Just think about how uncomfortable you would feel in only 15 seconds with an insufficient amount of oxygen. Endothelial cells become similarly disturbed with insufficient amounts of vitamins to support adequate production of NO. They become dysfunctional as rapidly as you would become alarmed if your oxygen supply was cut off. What happens is nothing short of amazing! Perfectly healthy cells become dysfunctional. The activity of NO Synthase enzymes is decreased, followed by a decrease in NO production. NO-deprived endothelial cells then become dysfunctional, making even less NO.

This vicious cycle can result in waking up the chronic degenerative diseases that are carried in our genes through hereditary factors. In other words, we become prone to develop the diseases that our ancestors had—or would have had if they lived long enough. Thus, GH should be treated as soon as it's suspected, by taking steps to foster homeostasis and slow down entropy.

"Apoptosis is an amazing thing," writes Dr. William Patrick Tansey in a landmark review in the July 24, 2004, edition of the *New England Journal of Medicine*, because "by endowing cells with the ability to kill themselves when they are dysfunctional, damaged, or malignant, nature allows the entire body and our life to be spared."

So you see, whether it's dysfunctional endothelial cells or wild cancer cells that are threatening to run amok, the signal is sent to initiate apoptosis in order to protect the rest of the body. Nature has determined that our sick cells must be replaced by vigorous new cells, so apoptosis—cellular suicide—is our evolutionary friend for survival. But this survival strategy comes at a price, because strong mechanisms must exist in our bodies to keep apoptosis inactive under normal conditions. Vitamins and minerals, especially antioxidants, play an invaluable role.

Dr. Tansey writes, "By its very nature, apoptosis demands that our normal, healthy cells always carry with them all the proteins required for their own cell death. In good times, these components must be tightly controlled to prevent premature cell death; however, this is only half the story. When the time comes for a cell to die, the safety mechanisms that were put in place must be removed . . . and quickly."

The signal for apoptosis, which can simply diminish the Spark of Life discovered by Dr. Murad, causes an *orderly* cascade of molecular and chemical destruction in the cells, not a chaotic three-ring circus. The *New England Journal of Medicine* review describes the situation rather eloquently: "Everything in the cell isn't simply going to hell."

Not surprisingly, the discovery of the orderly, apoptotic cascade of events has led scientists all over the world to concentrate on initiating or somehow accelerating the apoptosis cascade in order to destroy cancer cells—*by using drugs to trick cancer cells into committing suicide*.

The goal of **The Wellness Solution** is very different. It's a specific lifestyle plan directed at boosting NO to stop the signal for apoptosis from occurring in the first place—or to interrupt the orderly cascade if it's already begun. You now understand the molecular basis for helping to prevent and treat GH, by fostering homeostasis and decreasing entropy. Once again, we believe that identifying this abnormal condition can help stem the tide of chronic degenerative diseases in the modern world.

An Interesting Question

Was there ever a time when people didn't need to use vitamin and mineral supplements? After all, weren't our bodies designed to last in harmony with nature?

Yes, when our ancestors' diet consisted mostly of fruit, vegetables, and whole grains, with just small amounts of animal flesh and by-products.

Yes, when they hunted, gathered, fished, and farmed in the fields and the forests and on the oceans from sunup to sundown.

Yes, when the sunlight was not yet toxic because the ozone layer had not been depleted.

Yes, when the rain did not have acid in it because of environmental pollutants.

Yes, when the oceans, rivers, and drinking water were not yet contaminated.

Yes, in a time when the unremitting fear and worry generated by instantaneous reporting of frightening news from all over the world did not exist.

That was then.

But for now, we urge you to follow

The Wellness Solution

Thank you for having read this far in our book. You can now be sure that you know more about NO and GH than 99 percent of all the people in the world, because new medical discoveries, even those that win the Nobel Prize, take so long to be accepted. The best part is yet to come—that's called a paradigm shift, which is a brand-new viewpoint and mind-set for you that will forever determine the way you view the human body and especially your health destiny. It cannot completely be discovered or understood by you until you read the rest of this book. However, before you proceed, there is a question you should ask yourself: *Why should I trust and take the advice of the authors of this book?*

We believe the answer has to do with the importance of forming a therapeutic relationship with us, because knowledge is power only when you act upon it. This means you need to trust us. In return, we pledge that we will never betray your trust. In the practice of medicine, trust between physicians and patients is crucial to diagnose and treat the full range of diseases that we face today. Otherwise, what physicians call the "compliance factor," which is how much patients actually follow their physicians' advice, won't be satisfactory. And as you probably know, most patients don't exactly follow all their doctors' advice.

From reading the foreword, you already know about David Oliphant, including his successful track record of making profound ideas understandable to virtually everyone. It's also important for you to have more information about the physician co-authors to help you make the decision to comply with our prescription for your health. Compliance is crucial, and if you trust us, you will be much more likely to comply. Otherwise, compliance too often requires a wake-up call, such as a life-threatening event or a scary symptom like chest pain.

Any time you choose a doctor—whether in person or via a book—you should know about the doctor's training and accomplishments. Therefore, in next part of our book, "Meet the Doctors," we invite you to read a bit about our personal lives, along with a brief discussion about our accomplishments.

PART THREE

MEET THE DOCTORS

Edward A. Taub, M.D.

Please allow me to introduce myself. My name is Edward Taub. I've been a medical doctor for over 40 years. I'm a board-certified pediatrician, a family doctor, a medical teacher, and an author of six books on wellness and preventive medicine. I'm also QVC's Wellness Medical Doctor.

I am blessed to be living a wonderful life with a very special wife and family. It is my honor to share some of my personal story and credentials with you.

My parents were just teenagers, living in the Bronx, New York, when I was born. My mom was all of 16, and my dad was 17. My grandparents had fled from Russia and Hungary during World War I. They worked very hard in America—my grandmother was a seamstress, and my grandfather waited on tables in Manhattan's Lower East Side. They saved enough money to open a little candy store in east Manhattan.

Before kindergarten I spent my days in the candy store while my parents were working. I loved learning to read the comic books that were sold in the store, especially the "Illustrated Classics"—about 100 of them! The great novels—presented like comic books, with amazing illustrations—became so thoroughly embedded in my young mind that it actually helped me do extremely well with the tests required to gain admission to the best schools in New York City.

I graduated from the Bronx High School of Science at the young age of 15. While there, my unwavering love for the history and philosophy of science was born. I went to college at the State University of New York in Binghamton, on a New York Regents Scholarship. I spent equal time in college on literature and biology and gained acceptance to a fine postgraduate program in classical literature as well as a fine medical school. It was a very difficult decision to make, but I chose medicine— a very wise choice! I still very much enjoy reading great works of literature . . . and remember the "Illustrated Classics" very fondly.

I received my medical degree from the Upstate Medical Center in Syracuse, New York, in 1963 and headed west to California for my internship, where I have lived ever since. However, from 1964 to 1966, I proudly served as Lieutenant Commander in the United States Coast Guard, in charge of the outpatient clinic of U.S. Marine Hospital in Detroit. Also, from 1992 to 1995, I directed the Wellness Medicine Institute in Mt. Carmel, Illinois.

During my rotating internship at the Orange County General Hospital in California, I found myself thrown into the unnerving position of being largely responsible for the acute care of dozens of patients every day. Every two months I rotated from pediatrics to oncology to surgery to OB-GYN to geriatrics and, finally, the psychiatry wards.

My choice for a specialty was pediatrics, and I began my residency at the Los Angeles County–USC General Hospital (1966 to 1968). It made my experience as an intern look like kids stuff! Instead of being "largely" responsible for very sick patients, now I *was* responsible— for tiny preemies and sick newborns to children with meningitis, diabetes, leukemia, heart disease, kidney disease, liver disease, and much more, from tetanus to rattlesnake bites, while *also* being responsible for teaching the medical students and interns on my wards. As I reflect back now, this experience helped me develop a profound sense of a physician's responsibility for patient care and for teaching other physicians. This responsibility has always been the highest priority for me.

Several unforgettable phases in my practice as a physician have defined and focused my vision about health care. The first phase was devoted to caring for infants, children, and adolescents during my first two decades in medicine, when I specialized strictly in the practice of pediatrics. The first breath of life and the first smile that newborns shared with me, along with the imagination and courage of children with leukemia, diabetes, or congenital birth defects, taught me quite a different language than my medical books did. I learned that much of our capacity to be healthy and happy as adults depends on our ability to become fluent again in the child-like language of imagination and courage. Children taught me to under- stand how much we would benefit if we had more trust and hope.

I learned the full meaning of this lesson during the second phase of my career, when I spent over two decades being a family doctor, treating pa- tients of all ages. So many of my adult patients have been remarkable— not so much for the severity of their illnesses, but for the sheer magnitude of their determination to live life to the fullest extent possible.

I've written several books to share the lessons my patients taught me. One of the most endlessly fascinating aspects of medical practice is that patients have their own unique stories and personal feelings about their illnesses and ailments. Now I find myself more receptive and able to empathize with my patients' pain and suffering . . . understanding their worry and hurt. I have experienced their frustrations and triumphs, and the books I have written have been inspired by the trust and hope that my patients, especially the children, first taught me.

I'm very proud to tell you that I helped pioneer the wellness move- ment and founded the field of Integrative Medicine, combining good medical science with responsible self-care. I presented the initial paper on this subject to the Institute of Medicine in Washington, D.C., in 1982.

My mission is to help people *stay well in the first place*—or, if they are sick, to help them understand what is happening to them and what they can do about it. My previous books, especially *Balance Your Body, Balance Your Life,* which was made into a PBS television special, have given me an opportunity to spread my wellness message.

As QVC's Wellness Medical Doctor, I have the unique opportunity to practice Wellness Medicine on a grand scale on television in over 90 million homes. It's an enormous responsibility that requires me to constantly be researching current medical literature.

I'm very fortunate to have a loving wife, Anneli, who divides her time between painting, gardening, and coaxing me to lead a more balanced life, so I can practice what I preach.

For healthy nutrition and weight management, I depend on Anneli's cooking skills, which are on dramatic display in the wonderful recipe section of this book. For recreation, I love sailing. I'm part of the crew on a historic schooner called Curlew.

Please meet some more of my family. My son, Marc Taub, M.D., is an emergency department physician and director; my daughter, Lora Taub, Ph.D., is a university professor of communications; and my brother, Lanny Taub, M.D., is a pediatrician. Finally, my two grandchildren, Lucas and Leila, are exceptional.

Two titles were conferred upon me during my medical school graduation. The first one was that of "Doctor," when the dean handed me my diploma. The second title was conferred after I took the Hippocratic oath to serve my patients. Then, before man and God, I became a physician. I believe very strongly that God gives us all a special purpose in life. Mine was being a medical doctor.

Along the way in life, I've been privileged to work with Dr. Ferid Murad, who has made scientific discoveries of such profound dimensions that they will endure for as long as oxygen needs to delivered to human cells for life. My enduring friendship with David Oliphant is based on a lifetime of deep admiration, appreciation, and respect.

Thank you and stay well!

Edward A. Taub

Ferid Murad, M.D., Ph.D.

Please allow me to also introduce myself. My name is Ferid Murad. I'm a medical doctor, a board-certified internist, and the chairman of the University of Texas Medical School Department of Integrative Biology and Pharmacology. Also, I'm the director of the University of Texas Institute of Molecular Medicine.

It was a great honor to share the 1998 Nobel Prize in Medicine for the discovery that Nitric Oxide is the body's signaling molecule. It's a wonderful life I lead, with a wonderful family. It is my pleasure to share some of my life's personal stories with you.

My father and his family were shepherds in Albania. He left home when he was a teenager to sell candy in the Balkan countries, and he then immigrated to the United States, where he eventually became a very proud U.S. citizen. After working in the steel mills in Cleveland and Detroit, he settled in Chicago. Although he had less than a year of education, he learned to speak seven languages. My mother was born in Alton, Illinois. She went to grade school for several years before she quit so she could help her mother and younger siblings. My mom left home at age 17, in 1935, to marry my dad.

I was born a year later, at home, in their hot and small apartment over a bakery in Whiting, Indiana.

The childhood poverty of my parents and their minimal education did a lot to influence my education and career choices. We owned and took care of a small restaurant. When I was able to stand on a stool to reach the sink, I washed dishes.

Later, when I could see over the counter, I waited on tables and managed the cash register. This was my work throughout grade school and high school, every evening and on weekends. Dad worked 16 to 18 hours a day in the restaurant, while my mother put in similar hours between the restaurant and raising three children. They owned the building which housed our restaurant; it included sleeping rooms upstairs. Many of the tenants were old, and my mother would care for them and prepare their meals when they were sick. This helped me develop a sense of compassion and generosity for people that eventually influenced my career choice—Medicine. Working long and hard hours is my modus operandi. Besides my love for my family, I have a love affair with my profession, which gives me great enjoyment.

Growing up with considerable freedom and saving my tips from the restaurant helped support my career choice. This freedom principle that my parents allowed me to enjoy also applied to my religious choices. Dad was a Muslim, Mom a Baptist, and we were raised in a Catholic community. Subsequently, my brothers chose Catholicism when they married Catholic wives. In college, I chose to be baptized Episcopalian. Carol Ann, my wonderful wife of more than 40 years, is Presbyterian. Three of our daughters married fine Jewish and Catholic men. We are a loving, caring, intellectually interesting mixed bag!

Believe it or not, I was on the track and cross-country team in high school, as a long-distance runner. I also played football and basketball; however, I spent most of my time keeping the bench warm. Most of us played offense and defense in those days. My position was left guard, and I was 5 feet 11 inches and weighed 140 pounds. After three monsters ran over me, it was prudent for me to spend more of my energy in long-distance running. Now, my sport is golf, and like most weekend hackers, it's a struggle.

Throughout college, I waited tables, taught anatomy labs, and worked one or two jobs during summers to cover my expenses. In my junior year, I met Carol Ann Leopold, who became my wife. Was I a lucky guy! Our dates were primarily "study dates" at the library (the only thing I could afford). We were married in 1958 and progressed with our family: four girls, including a set of identical twins before I finished medical and graduate schools in 1965. Number five, our first boy, was born as I finished my medical residency in 1967. Fortunately, we didn't stop as planned after number four was born.

I was first in my class at the Case Western Reserve University Medical School in Cleveland, Ohio. Learning was purely a labor of love.

There was never any doubt in my mind about pursuing an academic career in medicine, research, and teaching.

To survive economically in medical school with so many children, moonlighting at the Cleveland Clinic was a must. I worked nights on the OB-GYN service, and my responsibilities included caring for mothers by providing pelvic exams as they progressed through labor, assisting in deliveries and Caesarian sections, then scrubbing tables and floors after each delivery. This job paid me $20 per night for 12 hours of work, from 7 p.m. to 7 a.m. I did that one or two nights per week for four years. However, in spite of the poor pay, I felt a huge amount of personal gratitude toward the people I helped.

Sometimes, the schedule required that I work all night and then attend a full day of classes the next day. This took me away from my family as often as four to five nights per week. My wife and children were very understanding. They grew up as wonderful children and adults in spite of my absence, thanks to my wife. Carol Ann is a devoted wife and mother.

It was a priority to spend several weeks each summer with my family. We took them camping all over the United States. My current fetish is my eight grandchildren, whom I try to spend as much time with as possible, undoubtedly due to my guilt as an absent father.

Massachusetts General Hospital was where I went for my internship and residency in internal medicine (1965–1967). What a wonderful experience that was, with some of the world's leading teachers, including the chief of medicine, Dr. Alex Leaf. There couldn't have been a better introduction to medicine. After my residency, I began my research career at the NIH Heart Institute; then the University of Virginia asked me to form a new clinical pharmacology division. I was 33 years old with five children.

Of the 105 research fellows and students I trained and collaborated with, many have become professors, chairmen, research directors, and division chiefs around the world. I view them as my offspring and keep in contact with most of them. *One of my proudest accomplishments is to have participated in the training of such fine scientists and to have influenced the careers of so many talented physicians.*

While it was difficult to leave friends and colleagues at the University of Virginia, where we conducted the first experiments with the biological effects of Nitric Oxide, I couldn't turn down the exciting opportunity that was offered to me by Stanford Medical School, where I served as the chief of medicine at the Veterans Hospital and acting chairman of the Department of Medicine and continued to supervise a large productive laboratory with trainees from all over the world.

After Stanford, I became a vice president at Abbott Laboratories, where I helped discover many novel drug targets and brought forward 24 new medical compounds for clinical trials for various diseases. When I left Abbott, I was supervising about 1,500 scientists and staff. I then co-founded a biotechnology company that focused on Alzheimer's disease.

In 1996, I was honored to be awarded the Albert Lasker Award for Basic Medical Research for "having advanced the fundamental understanding of biochemical mechanisms in cells." In 1997, I was appointed the chairman of the Department of Integrative Pharmacology at the University of Texas Medical School in Houston, where I am also the director of the Institute of Molecular Medicine. In 1998, I shared the Nobel Prize in Medicine for my work with Nitric Oxide. This brings me full circle. I'm back in the academic element again and love it! The freedom and intellectual environment of academic medicine, along with the bright young students and fellows I have the pleasure of working with, are so exciting. They are a daily joy for me.

I have spent the past 47 years in medicine and research with a variety of positions and responsibilities. I remain quite intrigued and excited with medicine and biology, how the body works, how cells communicate with one another, and how this information can lead to the development of important therapy.

Finally, I am pleased to be working and collaborating with Dr. Edward Taub and David Oliphant. They are very experienced and caring individuals who continue to reinforce my learning process.

Thank you for reading this!

Ferid Murad

PART FOUR

THE WELLNESS SOLUTION

We are only as young—or as old—as our endothelium. So even though most Americans are living longer, they're also getting sicker as they age because the endothelium is deteriorating. A sick endothelium cannot produce enough NO.

Whether we develop a chronic degenerative disease depends very much on our family histories, how long we live, and how well we take care of ourselves. For example, medical researchers have discovered that the carotid arteries of obese children who are as young as 7 years old are getting thick and stiff—arterial disease already related to endothelial sickness. Compared with kids of normal weight, obese kids were found to have higher blood pressure, inflamed arteries, higher cholesterol, and signs of diabetes. What a wake-up call!

Let's consider what may already be happening to these children and to the majority of adults by the age of 50. Be prepared for a shock, because over 100 million American adults are already suffering from chronic conditions such as heart disease, cancer, and diabetes, which are diet- and exercise-related conditions resulting from endothelial sickness. Indeed, the majority of American adults beyond the age of 50 probably already have significant endothelial sickness. The troubling evidence includes the fact that every one of us who is 55 years of age or older has a 90 percent chance of developing hypertension!

What in the world is going on? This mind-boggling trend is easier to understand if we consider the fact that humans have a life cycle just like all other living things. The human life cycle consists of our growing years, reproductive years, the years spent caring for our families, and finally, our end-of-life years. Mother Nature graciously forgives all sorts of unhealthy behaviors during our growing and reproductive years in order to help us cast our human DNA into future generations through our offspring.

After these years, however, our bodies break down according to patterns that are inscribed as genetic templates or blueprints in our DNA. These templates or blueprints of diseases are meant to remain dormant until the time that our natural biological clock sounds its alarm toward the end of our life cycle.

The problem in today's world is that the templates of diseases are emerging prematurely and with alarming frequency, due to the war being waged in our bodies by free radicals and because we are living so much longer. Although medical science creates diagnostic labels for each of the templates, all of them are at least partially triggered by NO deficiencies, which can trigger chronic degenerative diseases.

COMMON FORMS OF CHRONIC DEGENERATIVE DISEASES

Alzheimer's Disease	Herpes Infection
Arthritis	HIV
Asthma and Emphysema	Hypertension
Atherosclerosis	IBS
Autoimmune Disease	Leukemia, Lymphoma, Hodgkin's
Cancer	Chronic Liver Disease
Cardiovascular Disease	Chronic Kidney Disease
Cataracts	Macular Degeneration (AMD)
Crohn's Disease	Obesity
Chronic Fatigue Syndrome	Osteoporosis
Depression	Parkinson's Disease
Diabetes	Pulmonary Hypertension/Fibrosis
Fibromyalgia	Tuberculosis
GERD	Ulcerative Colitis

Reducing Your Risk of Disease

Although this book addresses the full range of chronic degenerative diseases, the advice is especially helpful in reducing your risk of cardiovascular disease because that is so preventable. For that reason, we will focus on what can be done right now to start reducing your risk.

Before we get into *The Wellness Solution*, let's be very clear about what we mean by a "risk factor." Again, a risk factor is something or some condition that can make you more susceptible to a health problem. Remember, the *Journal of the American Medical Association* featured a report that said about *90 percent* of patients with severe heart disease have one or more of the following risk factors:

- Obesity
- Sedentary Lifestyle
- Diabetes Mellitus
- High Cholesterol or Abnormal Blood Lipids
- High Blood Pressure
- Angina or Previous Heart Attack
- Chronic Stress
- Age Older than 50 Years
- Family History of Heart Disease
- Smoking or Substance Abuse

Now is the time to assess whether any of those risk factors apply to you. If so, then you are a great candidate for *The Wellness Solution*. Please take a moment to evaluate your individual cardiovascular risk level according to our analysis of the scientific research.

RISK LEVELS

Category One: If you have one of the listed risk factors, then your endothelium is probably already showing signs of sickness.

Category Two: If you have two or three of the listed risk factors, then your endothelium is probably moderately sick.

Category Three: If you have four or five of the listed risk factors, then your endothelium is probably very sick.

Category Four: If you have more than five of the listed risk factors, then your endothelium is probably too sick to produce enough NO to make your blood vessels relax so that your blood can flow normally to help avoid heart attacks, strokes, and many chronic diseases.

An honest assessment of your risk category should provide you with a very good idea about your level of endothelial health and your risk for disease. This is simply a commonsense approach to caring more conscientiously for your health and well-being. But take heart! The human body is so resilient that whatever risk category you are in, you can still promote endothelial health and take greater charge of your health destiny with the strategic guidelines of *The Wellness Solution*.

You should implement this health strategy in conjunction with whatever medical care is prescribed by your own medical doctor. Indeed, regular consultations with your physician are important. This is true especially for patients with hypertension who may require blood pressure medication. Also, patients with diabetes who need good supervision to control their blood glucose and all individuals with an increased risk of cardiovascular disease should discuss with their physician whether they are candidates for aspirin therapy or a statin drug to lower cholesterol. Finally, ask your physician for a C-reactive protein (CRP) blood test to check the level of inflammation in your arteries. If you are seeing a doctor, for whatever reason, he or she should be delighted that you are taking the initiative to reduce your risk of disease. Your doctor should support you wholeheartedly as you pursue this healthful strategy.

To sum up, our longevity might have increased over the last hundred years, but for many people the longevity will just be cosmetic, because conditions like Generalized Hypovitaminosis, obesity, smoking, substance abuse, a sedentary lifestyle, and chronic stress have combined to slowly but surely weaken their endothelium. Taking proactive steps to improve your endothelial health, right now, helps reduce your risk for heart disease and other chronic degenerative diseases. We believe the most pressing public health need today is promoting endothelial health by following *The Wellness Solution*.

THE WELLNESS SOLUTION

1. **Healthy Nutrition**

2. **Weight Management**

3. **Appropriate Amounts of Water**

4. **A Scientifically Balanced Vitamin and Mineral Nutrition System**

5. **Regular Exercise**

6. **No Smoking . . . No Excess Alcohol . . . No Substance Abuse**

7. **Stress Management . . . Along with Being a Good Person**

The Wellness Solution is designed to be an easy regimen for you to follow. However, we are fully aware that even the most brilliant recommendations will be valueless if they can't be easily followed.

We believe our recommendations are strong and sound, but we also know that they are only as good as your actions and compliance. Please keep on reading so you will continue to understand how to promote endothelial health by examining *The Wellness Solution* in more detail.

Healthy Nutrition

Just one fast-food meal can make your endothelial cells sick. Even if you are otherwise healthy, one fast-food meal reduces the ability of your blood vessels to function normally for several hours.

—John Cooke, M.D., Ph.D.,
Stanford University School of Medicine

Dr. Cooke's staggering news is based on a study of people who ate a single meal from a typical fast-food restaurant. Within two hours of consuming the meal, these individuals had almost a 50 percent decrease in the normal function of their endothelium! Dr. Cooke is the director of the Section of Vascular Medicine at Stanford University Medical School. His research demonstrates that extra fat shows up in our blood after consuming unhealthful food and inhibits the production of NO, which makes our endothelium sick. This becomes a very unhealthy, vicious cycle, because a sick endothelium makes even less NO.

Merely being overweight, for example, creates extra fat in the blood. This causes high blood pressure, diabetes, and many types of cancer, all of which make the endothelium sick. And again the ferocious cycle begins, because once the endothelium starts producing less NO, it gets even sicker.

The exciting news is that researchers, including Dr. Cooke, have discovered that a sick endothelium is resilient enough to improve with good care. So let's first discuss healthy nutrition and then weight management for endothelial wellness. Remember that the goal is optimal NO production.

Some Recommendations

For optimal NO production, we need to eat lots of fresh fruits and vegetables, whole grains, nuts, beans, and fish, along with generous amounts of olive or canola oil.

We suggest at least five servings of fresh fruits and veggies every day. Oatmeal and other whole grain cereals are especially recommended for breakfast, with soy milk. A small handful of nuts on most days is very healthy for you. Walnuts are probably the best. We also recommend eating fish at least two or three times a week. The healthiest types of fish are mackerel, herring, salmon, trout, sardines (canned in oil), and halibut, because they contain lots of essential omega-3 fatty acids. *Essential* means we need this type of fat to live.

Your body does not manufacture fatty acids by itself. You should limit eating other types of animal flesh to not more than three or four times a week—chicken and turkey are far healthier choices than beef or pork. Don't be fooled by advertising claiming that pork is the "other white meat."

Olive and canola oils are wonderful resources for endothelial wellness. Despite what you may think, it's important to eat fat because it's required for every cell in your body. Saturated fats are bad for your health, and unsaturated fats are good, in moderation. Eating too much saturated fat is a major cause of high cholesterol and of inflamed arteries and contributes to endothelial sickness. These are fats from animal products, and they are firm or get hard at room temperature. Don't let it confuse you, because it's relatively simple: the more saturated the fat, the harder the fat. Butter has more saturated fat than margarine.

Unsaturated fats come mostly from plant and fish sources and are much healthier than saturated fats. These fats are soft or liquid at room temperature. Nuts, olive oil, and canola oil contain mostly unsaturated fat. There are two major types of unsaturated fats: polyunsaturated (good) or monounsaturated (even better). Eating for a healthy endothelium requires a mixture of both types. Olive oil, canola oil, avocados, walnuts, peanuts, cashews, and almonds provide wonderful nutrition for our endothelium, because they contain mostly monounsaturated fat with less polyunsaturated fat.

The only types of fat worse for our endothelium than saturated fats are man-made trans fats. These awful fats are found in most fast foods and in snacks and baked goods that are commercially produced for mass consumption. Virtually all hamburger and fried chicken chains use trans fats in oil to fry food, as do most casual dining establishments. And Americans eat out a lot! According to the National Restaurant Association, 46 percent of the food dollar is spent eating outside the home. That means we are consuming a lot of trans fats.

How awful are trans fats? Well, they lower good cholesterol (HDL) and raise bad cholesterol (LDL) so aggressively that in the Harvard Nurses' Health Study, women who ate the most transfats were *50 percent* more likely to die of heart disease. Is there a more compelling reason to choose fresh fruits, nuts, vegetables, and whole grains over fast food and junk food, which not only cause obesity, but can kill you?

Healthy amounts of good protein are crucial for endothelial health. The actual meaning of the word *protein* is derived from the Greek word meaning "prime importance." Vegetable protein is healthier than animal protein, and soy protein seems to be the healthiest of all when it comes to promoting heart and blood vessel health. It seems difficult to get sufficient soy into our meals, but it's worth trying. Eating a whole grain cereal for breakfast, along with cold soymilk, is one way to start, and the edamame soybean recipe that follows later on makes a delicious appetizer, snack, or main course.

Many of the nutritional guidelines described above fit into what is generally known as a Mediterranean-style diet, since it's the traditional way of eating in France, Italy, Greece, Spain, and Portugal. People in these Mediterranean countries experience cardiovascular disease at strikingly lower rates than those in the United States. But it's wrong to think of this manner of eating as a *diet*—it's an entire wellness lifestyle. Two landmark studies and an accompanying editorial about the Mediterranean-style diet were published in the *Journal of the American Medical Association* in September 2004. The studies reinforce the notion that *"we are only as young—or as old— as our endothelium."*

The first study demonstrates that a healthy lifestyle is just as important as the Mediterranean way of eating, especially for people who are between 70 and 90 years old. The researchers followed 2,400 Western European men and women for 10 years and discovered that those following a Mediterranean-style diet and a wellness lifestyle had almost a two-thirds lower rate of death from *all causes*. The researchers conclude: "Therefore, a diet rich in plant foods, in combination with nonsmoking, moderate alcohol consumption, and at least 30 minutes of physical activity per day, is associated with a significantly lower mortality rate, even in old age."

The second study focuses on the use of a Mediterranean-style diet to treat the very prevalent Metabolic Syndrome. This syndrome, which affects about 25 percent of all American adults, includes high blood fats, high blood pressure, diabetes or prediabetes, and abdominal obesity, which are all signs of endothelial sickness. Abdominal obesity is defined as a waist circumference greater than 40 inches for men and greater than 35 inches for women. The researchers proved that the Mediterranean-style diet was a safe, effective treatment for people with Metabolic Syndrome. Eating this way reduces the risk of cardiovascular disease by improving endothelial health and stimulating NO production.

How effective was this eating lifestyle? It reduced the presence of Metabolic Syndrome's components by about 50 percent. That's nothing short of amazing! The researchers conclude that their findings "represent the first demonstration, to our knowledge, that a Mediterranean-style diet rich in whole grains, fruits, vegetables, legumes, walnuts, and olive oil might be effective in reducing both the prevalence of the Metabolic Syndrome and its associated cardiovascular risk." The study also suggests a real breakthrough in understanding the link between nutrition, endothelial health, and NO production.

In an editorial commenting on the significance of these studies, Drs. Eric B. Rimm and Myer J. Stampfer, respected Harvard physicians associated with the famous Harvard Nurses' Health Study, claim that the new information is a "call to action." A simple set of lifestyle practices can reduce the mortality rate among elderly individuals by nearly two-thirds! The doctors wisely observe: "As a society, the United States spends billions on chronic disease treatments and interventions for risk factors. Although these are useful and important, just a fraction of that investment to promote healthful lifestyles for primary prevention among individuals at all ages would yield greater benefit."

The Wellness Solution is an effective response to the Harvard physicians' call to action. Unfortunately, Americans' eating habits are not even close to the ideal of following a Mediterranean-style diet. To help you achieve a more healthful nutrition lifestyle, we would like to share some of our favorite personal recipes with you. It will be like a cookbook within our book. Please note that these recipes have been tested and approved by a chef trained at the famous Culinary Institute of America.

HEALTHFUL RECIPES

SALADS

Antipasto di Anneli

MAKES 4 SERVINGS

12 *stalks asparagus, steamed until tender, and halved*

1 *12-ounce jar artichoke hearts in water, drained*

1 *red bell pepper, sliced in thin strips*

1 *red onion, thinly sliced*

1 *cup sun-dried tomatoes (softened in a bowl of hot water, drained, and chopped)*

1 *8-ounce can Kalamata olives in water, drained*

8 *leaves fresh basil, chopped coarsely*

2 *tablespoons olive oil*

2 *tablespoons balsamic vinegar*

2 *tablespoons lemon juice*

^{1}/2 cup shaved Asiago cheese

pepper to taste

NOTE: To soften sun-dried tomatoes, place them in a bowl of scalding water and set aside for 15 to 20 minutes. Drain and chop.

1. On a large platter or serving plate, arrange asparagus, artichoke hearts, bell pepper, and onion.
2. Top with sun-dried tomatoes, olives, and basil.
3. Mix together olive oil, balsamic vinegar, and lemon juice. Drizzle over vegetables.
4. Top antipasto with Asiago cheese and season to taste with pepper.

Traditional Italian antipasto salads are so high in fat and calories. The vegetables are drenched in oil and soggy with layers of processed meats. This low-fat, vegetarian variety brings out the best flavors of an antipasto. It's filled with Italian delicacies, such as artichoke hearts and sumptuous olives, but goes light on the high-fat cheeses and unhealthful oils.

Caesar Salad

MAKES 2 SERVINGS

We feel that this recipe has all the goodness of a traditional Caesar salad without the unhealthful traditional raw egg.

1/2 *cup Parmesan cheese, grated*

1 *tablespoon low-fat plain yogurt*

4 *garlic cloves, minced*

juice of half a lemon

1 *tablespoon Worcestershire sauce*

1/2 *tablespoon Dijon mustard*

pepper and salt or salt-substitute to taste

8 *leaves romaine lettuce, washed and torn*

1. To prepare the dressing, combine the first six ingredients in a medium-sized mixing bowl and whisk well. Season dressing to taste with pepper.
2. Pour dressing over lettuce and toss to coat leaves thoroughly.

There are endless healthful variations on this timeless classic. Unfortunately, most lack the flavor of a true Caesar salad. This variation tastes just like a Caesar salad is supposed to taste!

Tomato Mozzarella Salad

MAKES 2 SERVINGS

We can actually eat this salad as a main course. With fresh bread for soaking up the zesty vinaigrette, it is a substantial and healthy meal.

2 *tablespoons pine nuts, toasted (walnuts are suitable, too)*

2 *cloves garlic, mashed*

$1/2$ *tablespoon olive oil*

$1/2$ *cup arugula, washed and torn in bite-sized pieces*

5 *leaves romaine lettuce, washed and torn in bite-sized pieces*

$1/2$ *tablespoon balsamic vinegar*

pepper to taste

1 *tablespoon raisins, soaked in water for 10 minutes*

2 *large tomatoes, cut in wedges*

8 *ounces low-fat mozzarella cheese, cut in $1/4$-inch slices*

1. Combine nuts with garlic and olive oil. Spread on a foil-covered baking sheet and toast in a 350-degree oven for 5 minutes, until golden brown. (Keep a close eye on this, because it browns quickly.)

2. In a large bowl, toss greens with vinegar and season to taste with pepper. Stir in raisins and toasted nuts.

3. On a platter, arrange tomato wedges and cheese slices around the tossed greens.

4. Serve with crunchy Italian bread or fresh baguettes.

The fresh and tangy tastes of this salad make a delicious meal in itself. Wonderfully light and crisp and easy to prepare, this salad is full of energy and protein. Pine nuts come from the cones of the stone pine and have a deep, rich flavor. Combined with low-fat mozzarella, this light salad packs a protein punch. For a lively variation, substitute small bits of apple for the raisins.

Anneli's Tomato Salad

MAKES 4 SERVINGS

This is a simple yet sensational salad. The freshest vine-ripened tomatoes will create the most flavorful salad.

8 *medium tomatoes, cut in small wedges*

1 *tablespoon rice vinegar (seasoned)*

$^1/_2$ *small onion, minced*

1 *tablespoon parsley, finely chopped*

1 *teaspoon sugar*

black pepper to taste

$^1/_2$ *teaspoon salt or salt-substitute*

1. Place tomato wedges in a medium bowl. Set aside.
2. In another bowl, mix together vinegar, onion, parsley, sugar, pepper, and salt or salt-substitute, beating well with a fork.
3. Pour mixture over tomatoes and toss lightly.
4. Try serving with veggie burgers and fresh corn.

Tomatoes are a versatile fruit used as a vegetable, high in vitamin C. To keep tomatoes fresh and flavorful, do not refrigerate them. This may seem counter-intuitive, but it's true. The cold refrigerator not only destroys a fresh tomato's flavor, it may destroy its vitamins. When buying tomatoes, buy only as many as you can use in the next three or four days. The extra trip to the store or farmer's market will be well worth it. Rice vinegar gives this salad loads of flavor without loading it with the fat of traditional salad dressings. This salad is virtually fat-free.

Fast Green Bean Salad

MAKES 2 SERVINGS

Savory, tasty, and tangy, this salad is a treat for the taste buds and so easy to prepare. Use fresh green beans if they are in season.

1 *14-ounce can French-cut green beans, drained (or fresh, if available)*

1 *tablespoon onion, finely grated*

1 *tablespoon parsley, finely chopped*

1 *tablespoon white vinegar*

$^1/_4$ teaspoon salt or salt-substitute

$^1/_2$ teaspoon Maggi

dash each of pepper and sugar

1 *tablespoon canola oil*

1. Drain the water from the beans and empty them into a bowl. Add the remaining ingredients and mix well, so that all the beans are coated with dressing.

Green beans are a high-fiber vegetable. A great, tasty way to get most of the nutritional fiber you need in a day is to enjoy this salad. This is quick and simple but has a distinct flavor, thanks to the blend of Maggi, pepper, and sugar. Maggi is a condiment which has a nutty taste and is widely used in Germany. It's also great for soups, instead of salt. Look for Maggi in the gourmet foods or condiment section at your market.

SAUCE

Simple Fresh Tomato Sauce

MAKES 2 SERVINGS

The best tomato sauce comes from the freshest ingredients.

$1/2$ *tablespoon olive oil*

1 *small onion, finely diced*

3 *cloves garlic, crushed*

1 *small carrot, peeled and shredded*

6 *ripe tomatoes, diced*

2 *tablespoons fresh basil, chopped*

pepper and salt or salt-substitute to taste

dash of sugar

1. Heat oil in a medium-sized pan and add onion, garlic, and carrot. Sauté over medium heat for about 8 minutes, until onion is soft, but not brown.
2. Add the tomatoes and basil and simmer on low heat for 15 minutes, stirring often. Season to taste with pepper, sugar, and salt or salt-substitute.

This sauce is low fat, and served with a plate of steaming pasta. This makes a low-fat, high-energy meal. Select fresh tomatoes carefully. Look for bruises or soft spots. Choose vine-ripened tomatoes if available. When basil is not in season, or for variation, use fresh parsley in the recipe. A little sugar helps bring out the taste in tomatoes. For a pure, healthy, and easy-to-prepare tomato sauce, this recipe can't be beat. Lycopene gives tomatoes their red color, and it is probably the substance that decreases prostate cancer significantly in men who eat lots of tomato sauce.

SOUPS

Cold Tsatziki Soup

MAKES 4 SERVINGS

Smooth and cool, this authentic Greek soup comes together in hardly any time. It's perfect for a light lunch and tastes even better on the second day.

2 *cucumbers, peeled and coarsely grated*

pepper and salt or salt-substitute to taste

1 *pint low-fat plain yogurt*

juice of half a lemon

1 *garlic clove, mashed*

2 *cups water*

2 *tablespoons fresh mint, finely chopped*

1. Place cucumbers in a medium bowl and season to taste with salt-substitute and pepper. Set aside.
2. In another bowl, mix yogurt with lemon juice, garlic, and water.
3. Combine the cucumbers and yogurt mixture, add mint leaves, and stir well.

This soup is perfect for a hot summer day. The cool and crisp flavors of cucumber and mint are delicious and refreshing. Fresh mint gives this soup its distinct taste. Mint is easy to grow. If you don't have a garden, even a small container on the windowsill will produce amazing results. If mint is too strong for your taste, substitute fresh parsley for a more subtle soup.

Savory Green Bean Soup

MAKES 4 SERVINGS

This soup is hearty and healthful, the perfect meal in itself.

> 5 *cups water*
>
> 1 *teaspoon summer savory herb*
>
> 3 *cups green beans*
>
> 2^1/2 *tablespoons canola oil (* ^{1}/2 *tablespoon for browning onions,*
>
> 2 *tablespoons for browning flour)*
>
> 2 *medium onions, finely diced*
>
> 3 *tablespoons all-purpose flour*
>
> 1 *tablespoon vinegar*
>
> 2 *teaspoons sugar*
>
> 2 *teaspoons salt or salt-substitute*
>
> 1 *pound wide egg noodles*

1. Add summer savory to water and boil. Add beans and cook for 20 minutes.
2. While beans cook, heat ^{1}/2 tablespoon canola oil in a small skillet and sauté onions until brown. Transfer onions to a small bowl and set aside. In the same skillet, heat 2 tablespoons canola oil and add flour, stirring constantly to avoid clumping. Cook flour until golden brown and barely smoking. Watch carefully, flour turns from brown to burned very quickly!
3. Add onions and flour to the beans and water, and stir. Add vinegar, sugar, and salt or salt-substitute, and let simmer for 15 minutes.
4. While soup simmers, boil water for noodles. Cook noodles *al dente*. Serve soup hot, over noodles.

Garden-fresh green beans are the key to this flavorful soup. Greens picked from the garden are loaded with life energy. Look for a local farmer's market for the freshest beans available. If fresh beans aren't possible, frozen or canned beans are a good alternative. If you have children, involve them in the preparations—they love the popping sound that beans make when they break off the ends!

Fresh Vegetable Broth

MAKES ABOUT 5 CUPS

Here is the perfect way to use up vegetables in the fridge. This broth gives Vegetable Risotto a wonderful flavor.

2 *large carrots, sliced*

1 *large onion, sliced*

2 *celery stalks (outer), sliced*

a few celery leaves

a few parsley stems

2 *sprigs each of fresh thyme and marjoram*

2 *bay leaves*

3 *garlic cloves, crushed with the side of a knife*

a strip of lemon peel

10 *black peppercorns*

6 *cups water*

1. Put all ingredients in a large saucepan. Bring to a boil, then reduce the heat, cover the pan, and simmer until vegetables are just soft but not mushy—about 45 minutes. Let cool.

2. Strain broth through a sieve into a large container, pressing the solids to extract as much liquid as possible. Keep covered in the refrigerator. Use broth within four days.

Vegetable broth is simple and satisfying to make. Homemade is much healthier, and lower in sodium, than store-bought broth. You will taste the difference!

Broccoli Soup with Walnuts

MAKES 4 SERVINGS

This is a favorite autumn or winter soup. It is the perfect overture to a good meal, or a perfect meal in itself.

1 *medium onion, chopped*

4–5 *cups fresh broccoli, stems sliced and florets separated*

1 *tablespoon butter*

1 *cup vegetable bouillon or water*

1 *cup milk or plain soy or rice milk*

$1/4$ *cup half-and-half*

3 *tablespoons walnuts, chopped and toasted*

pepper and salt or salt-substitute to taste

1. In a large pot, sauté onion and broccoli in butter for 5 minutes.
2. Add bouillon (or water) and milk and simmer gently for 30 minutes, or until broccoli is tender.
3. Transfer to food processor or blender, puree until smooth, and return to pot.
4. Add half-and-half and walnuts. Season to taste with pepper and salt or salt-substitute.

This soup provides plentiful amounts of fiber to your diet. Broccoli and nuts are both high in fiber. Fiber helps remove excess cholesterol from the blood and thus helps keep your heart healthy. Broccoli may be the most maligned vegetable, but it is also one of the most healthful vegetables you can eat. Broccoli is loaded with compounds that help protect against cancer, as well as vitamin C and beta-carotene. Nuts are wonderful for your health when eaten regularly and in moderation. The monounsaturated fat and vitamin E in nuts help protect against heart disease.

Chicken Soup with Cabbage

MAKES 4 SERVINGS

This soup will fill your kitchen with a warm aroma. This recipe combines our favorite cabbage soup with chicken soup—a perfect marriage of flavors and traditions.

6 *cups water*

4 *skinless chicken breast fillets, sliced*

1 *small leek, cut in $^1/_2$-inch chunks*

2 *carrots, peeled and cut in 2-inch chunks*

1 *celery root, peeled and cut in $^1/_2$-inch chunks*

1 *bay leaf*

1 *small Savoy cabbage, cut in small pieces*

$^1/_4$ *cup chives, cut very thin (optional)*

$^1/_4$ *cup parsley, chopped*

pepper and salt or salt-substitute to taste

1. Bring water to a boil; add chicken and leek. Cover and cook on medium heat for about 30 minutes.
2. Add carrots, celery root, bay leaf, and cabbage. Cover and cook on low heat for another 30 minutes.
3. Just before serving, add parsley or chives, season to taste with pepper and salt or salt-substitute.
3. Serve over rice or just with some fresh crusty bread.
4. Remember to remove the bay leaf prior to eating the soup.

Wintertime is for soups, and this one is filled with hearty vegetables and chicken. Leftovers make a more flavorful soup the following day, and the broth can be used in many other recipes.

APPETIZERS

Edamame

MAKES 4–6 SERVINGS

When it comes to soy, edamame is the real thing! It's pronounced *eh-duh-MAH-may*, and it can be served as an appetizer or as an entrée. It's also a great breakfast, lunch, or dinner, all by itself.

1 *16-ounce package of frozen shelled soybeans*

1/4 cup olive oil (more if needed)

1 *large onion, peeled and finely chopped*

5 *garlic cloves, minced*

1/2 cup raisins

zest of 1 lemon

juice of 1 lemon

3 *sprigs fresh rosemary or thyme or 1 teaspoon dried herbs of Provence*

pepper and salt or salt-substitute to taste

1. Blanch soybeans, following directions on the package. Remove from heat and drain. While soybeans cook, heat olive oil in a pan. Add onions and sauté until golden brown. Add garlic for the last 5 minutes and also sauté until golden brown.
2. Pour cooked beans into a medium casserole dish. Add onions-garlic mixture. Add raisins, zest of lemon, lemon juice, pepper, and salt or salt-substitute. Stir together well. Layer sprigs of rosemary or thyme on top (or substitute herbs of Provence).
3. Put uncovered casserole dish in oven preheated to 375 degrees and bake for 15 minutes.

Serve warm or at room temperature. Try it with some crusty bread. The great taste, ease of preparation, and excellent nutrient value make this a wonderful soybean dish.

Portobello Appetizer

MAKES 4 SERVINGS

This is a wonderful appetizer. For a side dish, the rich flavors complement a crisp Caesar salad. It makes a great sandwich . . . with a little lettuce and tomato!

2 *tablespoons olive oil*

2 *large portobello mushrooms, stems removed, sliced thin*

2 *tablespoons balsamic vinegar*

pepper and salt or salt-substitute to taste

^{1}/2 *tablespoon fresh thyme, chopped*

1 *teaspoon fresh rosemary, chopped (substitute 3 teaspoons dried Italian herbs, if fresh herbs unavailable)*

2 *garlic cloves, peeled*

^{1}/2 *cup Parmesan cheese, grated*

1. In a medium skillet, heat 1 tablespoon oil and sauté portobellos until deep brown. Drain on a paper towel.
2. Arrange mushrooms on a plate, sprinkle with balsamic vinegar, pepper, salt or salt-substitute.
3. In the same skillet, combine chopped herbs and garlic and add 1 tablespoon olive oil. Mix well. Cook for 5 minutes on low heat.
4. Drizzle herb mixture over mushrooms.
5. Sprinkle mushrooms with Parmesan.
6. Serve mushrooms alone or on a baguette with sprigs of arugula and sliced tomatoes.

Rich, plump portobellos are our favorite variety of mushrooms. Once found only in specialty stores, they are now common in most supermarket produce sections.

Mock Chopped Liver

MAKES 6 SERVINGS

Chopped liver fans will rave about this healthy, low-fat variation of a traditional pâté. This recipe captures all the strong flavors of the original classic, but is much lower in fat and completely vegetarian.

$1/2$ *pound green beans, chopped in bite-sized pieces*

$3/4$ *pound mushrooms, chopped*

1 *small onion, peeled and finely chopped*

1 *teaspoon canola oil*

$1/4$ *cup walnuts, chopped*

pepper and salt or salt-substitute to taste

$1/4$ *cup water*

1. Sauté green beans, mushrooms, and onion in oil over medium-high heat for 10 minutes.
2. Pour mixture into food processor bowl, add remaining ingredients, and blend until creamy.
3. Chill and serve on a bed of lettuce with raw vegetables.

Thanks to creative cooking, snacking before dinner continues to be fun and healthy. Giving a dinner party? Going to a potluck? This is an excellent, easy-to-prepare, low-fat appetizer that will please vegetarians and nonvegetarians alike. For variation, this can be spread on bread for a delicious vegetarian sandwich.

French Salmon Spread

MAKES 4 SERVINGS

Many fans of French cuisine have had to give up their favorite French dishes because they do not accommodate a low-fat lifestyle. Over the years, we have learned to transform traditionally rich French recipes into low-fat, high-energy variations that still maintain their distinctly French flavor.

1 *tablespoon mustard (preferably Dijon)*

1 *tablespoon olive oil*

3 *ounces smoked salmon, finely chopped*

1 *tablespoon onion, minced (optional)*

1 *tablespoon greens of spring onion, finely chopped (chives can be substituted)*

pepper and salt or salt-substitute to taste

1. Mix mustard with oil until creamy.
2. Add salmon, onion, greens of spring onion or chives; season to taste with salt-substitute and pepper and mix well. Refrigerate for several hours before serving.
3. Simply tear off hunks of baguette and enjoy, or toast slices and top with spread.

Americans love appetizers. Unfortunately, most appetizers are high in fat and filled with meat. This dish is borrowed from the French and transformed into an intensely appetizing, but not sinfully fattening spread. Traditional rillettes are served throughout France, made of pork or rabbit. In this dish, salmon is substituted for a lighter, healthier spread, with terrific taste. If smoked salmon is unavailable, substitute another variety of smoked fish.

Hearty Garlic Spread

MAKES 1¹⁄₂ CUPS

This delicious spread earns its name because garlic truly is good for your heart. This is staple fare in the Mediterranean and the French countryside, combined with their zest for life. No wonder people from both areas have such low rates of heart disease! Traditionally, the spread is served to flavor crusty bread.

1 *cup silken tofu, firm*

6 *cloves garlic, peeled*

1 *tablespoon lemon juice*

1 *tablespoon olive oil*

pepper and salt or salt-substitute and pepper to taste

1. Combine all ingredients in a food processor and blend until smooth. Season to taste with pepper and salt or salt-substitute.
2. Refrigerate until serving in an airtight container; freshness lasts up to a week.

Peeling garlic can be frustrating if you don't know this simple trick: Place single cloves on a cutting board or counter. With the flat side of a large wooden spoon or a wide chef's knife, smash them. The peel just falls away. Garlic is wonderful for your health. Scientific studies have shown its preventive value in warding off bacteria, viruses, fungi, and other organisms that cause human disease. Chemicals in garlic also protect the heart. Researchers have shown that garlic has a cholesterol-lowering effect, reduces blood pressure, and can help prevent blood clots. Enjoy this as a dip for raw or steamed vegetables, or as a zesty sandwich spread.

SIDE DISHES

Stuffed Cucumbers Nany

MAKES 4 SERVINGS

Some friends introduced us to this savory dish. It's light, but surprisingly filling.

1 *cup brown rice*

2 *cups water*

1 *8-ounce package low-fat cream cheese*

2 *tablespoons raisins*

pepper and salt or salt-substitute to taste

5 *medium cucumbers, peeled, halved lengthwise, and seeded*

1 *8-ounce jar of simple tomato sauce or fresh tomato sauce*

1. Cook brown rice according to directions on package, but 10 minutes less than required cooking time.
2. Drain rice and mix with cream cheese and raisins. Pepper and salt or add salt-substitute to taste.
3. Fill half of the cucumbers with the rice mixture. Top each stuffed cucumber with another half and secure with toothpick.
4. Place stuffed cucumbers in a casserole dish.
5. Pour simple tomato sauce over stuffed cucumbers. Cover and bake for 45 minutes at 300 degrees.

We love vegetables in their natural, raw, fresh state. When we cook them, we favor recipes that draw out the naturally delicious flavors. It's easy to overcook vegetables and destroy not only their flavor, but their nutritional value. This delicious dish combines the cool taste of cucumbers with the sweetness of raisins and nutty taste of brown rice.

Roasted Vegetables

MAKES 2 SERVINGS

While these vegetables roast in a balsamic marinade, your kitchen will become remarkably fragrant. The vinegar draws out the vegetables' subtle flavors. Vegetables never tasted so good!

$^1/_2$ tablespoon balsamic vinegar

$1^1/_2$ tablespoons extra virgin olive oil

1 teaspoon salt or salt-substitute

1 tablespoon rosemary

1 cup mushrooms, halved

1 cup green beans, broken in half

1 medium onion, sliced

1 medium sweet potato, peeled and cut in large chunks

1 large carrot, peeled and cut in large chunks

5 cloves garlic, peeled

1. Preheat oven to 450 degrees.
2. Prepare marinade in a large bowl, combining vinegar, oil, salt-substitute, and rosemary.
3. Add vegetables, mushrooms, onions, and garlic to the marinade and coat evenly.
4. Spread vegetables out in a shallow baking pan and pour marinade on top.
5. Roast vegetables for 35 to 40 minutes (or until sweet potato is soft), stirring occasionally. Vegetables are done when they are a warm brown, caramel-like color.

There's nothing more delicious than the flavor of roasted fresh vegetables. Roasting vegetables brings out their naturally sweet juices.

Very Veggie Burgers

MAKES 10 PATTIES

1 *tablespoon canola oil*

$^1/_2$ *pound mushrooms, quartered*

1 *small onion, diced*

2 *tablespoons walnuts or sunflower seeds*

1 *large carrot, coarsely grated*

1 *tablespoon apple, peeled and grated*

1 *teaspoon marjoram*

pepper and salt or salt-substitute to taste

1 *cup green beans, cooked to crisp tender*

1 *cup Garbanzo beans, drained*

1 *tablespoon tahini or peanut butter*

1 *tablespoon Worcestershire sauce*

3 *tablespoons bread crumbs*

1 *egg white*

1. Heat oil in a large skillet. Add mushrooms, onion, nuts, carrot, apple, and marjoram. Sauté until mushrooms appear golden brown. Add pepper and salt or salt-substitute to taste.
2. Transfer vegetables to medium-sized bowl and add green beans, garbanzos, tahini or peanut butter, Worcestershire sauce, and bread crumbs.
3. Combine everything well and put in a food processor. Pulse 3 or 4 times. Mixture should be a coarse consistency. Mix in egg white. Form into palm-sized patties.
4. Bake on a nonstick baking sheet at 450 degrees for 15 minutes; flip and bake another 15 minutes. Or fry to golden brown in a skillet lightly coated with canola oil.

We searched the world for the best veggie burger. Some taste too much like soy, some have a gummy texture, some simply fall apart! Veggie burgers are a healthy alternative to hamburgers, but unless they're pleasurable to eat and tasty, why would anyone switch? Some veggie burgers try too hard to resemble hamburgers. That's not our goal with this recipe; this is a healthy and delicious low-fat burger sure to win over the toughest skeptics! Try these burgers on fresh sourdough bread or whole-wheat buns.

ENTREES

Farfalle with Beans and Tuna

MAKES 4 SERVINGS

This is a perfect dish to prepare when you have unexpected guests. It's simple, but delicious and can be enjoyed year-round.

1 *tablespoon olive oil*

1 *large onion, finely diced*

4 *cloves garlic, mashed*

2 *tablespoons Vermouth (optional)*

8 *fresh tomatoes, peeled and diced, or 1 28-ounce can crushed tomatoes*

1 *10-ounce package frozen lima beans, defrosted*

1 *teaspoon sugar*

pepper and salt or salt-substitute to taste

1 *tablespoon oregano*

1 *can tuna in water, drained and cut into small chunks*

1 *pound farfalle (bowtie pasta)*

1. Heat olive oil in large pot. Add onion and garlic and sauté until translucent. Add vermouth.
2. Add tomatoes, beans, sugar, and oregano. Season to taste with pepper and salt or salt-substitute. Cook on medium-low heat for 15 minutes.
3. Mix tuna into sauce and simmer for about 3 minutes, until tuna is just warm.
4. While sauce is simmering, cook pasta al dente and mix together with sauce; serve.

This dish proves there are delicious ways to eat high-protein meals without relying on high-fat red meat. Pasta, beans, and tuna combine to create a dish packed with energy, but low in fat.

Vegetable Risotto

MAKES 2 SERVINGS

Look for the freshest, most tender stalks of asparagus.

2 *cups trimmed asparagus tips*

3 *cups water*

1 *tablespoon olive or canola oil*

2 *shallots, chopped (about $^1/_4$ cup)*

1 *garlic clove, minced*

1$^1/_2$ *cups short-grain or Arborio rice*

vegetable broth recipe (see "Fresh Vegetable Broth" under SOUPS)

pinch of saffron threads (optional)

strip of lemon peel

1 *tablespoon lemon juice*

2 *cups sliced button mushrooms*

8 *sun-dried tomatoes packed in oil, well drained and chopped*

$^1/_2$ *cup chopped walnuts or cashews, toasted*

salt or salt-substitute and freshly ground black pepper

roughly chopped flat-leaf parsley and large shavings of Asiago cheese (optional) for garnish

1. Put asparagus in small saucepan of boiling water and cook until barely tender (2 to 3 minutes). Drain and reserve liquid. Refresh asparagus in ice water and set aside.

2. Heat oil in heavy saucepan. Add shallots and garlic; sauté 2 to 3 minutes. Stir in rice and cook 3 minutes, stirring occasionally.

3. Add enough vegetable broth to the reserved asparagus cooking liquid to make 3 cups. Add to the pan of saffron threads (if using) and lemon peel and juice. Bring to a boil, then reduce heat, cover, and simmer 10 minutes.

4. Add mushrooms and sun-dried tomatoes and cook, covered, until rice is tender —another 10 minutes. Stir in asparagus and nuts for the last few minutes of cooking.

5. Remove lemon peel, season to taste, and transfer to a warm dish. Sprinkle with chopped parsley and shavings of Asiago cheese (if using). Serve risotto at once.

Risotto is wonderfully creamy Italian rice. This dish takes a little longer to cook, but it is worth the extra time. You can substitute an endless variety of ingredients in this recipe.

Eggplant Rollatini

MAKES 4 SERVINGS

Thanks to some magnificent chefs, this delicious and healthy meal is low in calories and fat. For variety, we sometimes substitute fresh garden zucchini for eggplant.

$2/3$ *cup bread crumbs*

1 *tablespoon Parmesan cheese*

$1/4$ *teaspoon EACH dried ground basil, rosemary, parsley, and thyme*

$3/4$ *cup part-skim ricotta cheese*

1 *pound eggplant, cut into 12 slices, about $1/4$-inch thick*

1 *cup tomato sauce*

2 *tablespoons grated part-skim mozzarella cheese*

4 *ounces spaghetti or linguini*

1. Preheat oven to 350 degrees. Combine bread crumbs, Parmesan cheese, and half of herbs in small bowl; set aside.
2. In small bowl, mix remaining half of herbs into ricotta cheese and set aside.
3. Steam eggplant slices until pliable, about 3 to 5 minutes.
4. Lay each eggplant slice in crumbs, patting to be assured the coating will stick.
5. Spoon 1 tablespoon of ricotta cheese mixture near edge of each slice of eggplant and roll to form a tube.
6. Arrange eggplant rolls in shallow 8-inch by 11-inch baking dish. Sprinkle extra crumbs over them and top evenly with tomato sauce and mozzarella cheese. Bake until heated through, about 30 minutes.
7. While rollatini are baking, cook pasta, drain, and divide evenly among 4 plates.
8. Place 3 eggplant rollatini over pasta and serve immediately.

Eggplant is a staple of Italian cooking. In Italy, it's rarely fried, as it is here in the States. In this low-fat recipe (only 8 grams of fat per serving), the unique flavor of eggplant is enhanced with Italian herbs and tomatoes.

Asparagus Chicken

MAKES 4 SERVINGS

The appealing and unusual flavors of this dish consistently draw raves from family and friends. Delicate asparagus and mushrooms are drizzled with capers and lemon juice.

1^1/2 tablespoons canola oil

1 onion, finely chopped

2 cups mushrooms, sliced

2 whole skinless chicken breasts, cut into chunks (for vegetarian version, 1 lb. tofu)

3 tablespoons all-purpose flour

1 cup water

2 pounds fresh asparagus tips or 1 15-ounce can (save liquid)

2 tablespoons capers

juice of half a lemon

^{1}/2 tablespoon sugar

^{1}/2 tablespoon salt or salt-substitute and ^{1}/2 teaspoon pepper

2 cups basmati rice

4 cups water

1 tablespoon fresh parsley, chopped

1. Heat oil in medium pot and sauté onions until translucent. Add mushrooms and sauté until they turn light brown.
2. Add chicken and sauté until it appears white on all sides, about 10 minutes.
3. Sprinkle flour over chicken and stir well. Add water, asparagus and its juice, capers, lemon juice, pepper, sugar, and salt or salt-substitute. Cover and cook on low heat for 35 to 40 minutes, stirring occasionally.
4. In the meantime, cook basmati rice in water; follow directions on package.
5. Serve the asparagus chicken mixture over rice and sprinkle it with parsley.

The festivity of traditional German cooking is captured in this low-fat chicken dish. Capers and asparagus add unmistakable flavor. Try serving over halved puff pastry shells. This entrée is easily transformed into a vegetarian meal by substituting tofu for chicken.

Turkey Meatloaf

MAKES 4 SERVINGS

We have taken the high-fat American standard meatloaf and turned it into a healthful, low-fat meal—not your average ho-hum meatloaf!

$1/4$ *cup diced onion*

$3/4$ *pound ground skinless turkey breast*

$3/4$ *cup dry whole-wheat bread crumbs*

1 *egg white*

pinch of salt or salt-substitute

pinch of black pepper

$1/2$ *cup tomato sauce*

$1^1/2$ *teaspoons Worcestershire sauce*

1. Preheat oven to 350 degrees. Lightly spray baking sheet or loaf pan with nonstick vegetable coating and set aside.
2. Combine all ingredients in large bowl and mix well.
3. Form meat into loaf shape on baking sheet or put in loaf pan. Bake about 40 minutes or until loaf is firm to the touch.

If you and your family are making the transition away from red meat to a more vegetarian-based diet, this is the perfect meal! Turkey is much lower in fat than red meat. In fact, one serving of this meatloaf has only 4 grams of fat.

Chicken Goulash

MAKES 4 SERVINGS

We created a healthier version of beef goulash, so enjoy this wonderful dish!

2 tablespoons canola oil

2 medium onions, diced

2 skinless chicken breast fillets, cut into 2-inch chunks

16 ounces of mushrooms (brown, if available), cut in half

4 cloves garlic, sliced

1 tablespoon tomato paste

4 cups water

$^1/_2$ cup beer (optional)

1 teaspoon sugar

1 teaspoon paprika

pepper and salt or salt-substitute to taste

1 pound wide noodles

1. Heat oil in a large pot and add onions. Sauté until golden.
2. Add chicken. Stir frequently until chicken is golden brown, being careful not to burn.
3. Add mushrooms and garlic. Stir well. Cook for 10 minutes.
4. Add tomato paste and stir well for about 5 minutes.
5. Turn heat to medium/low. Slowly begin adding water, 1 cup at a time (also add beer, if using). Let each cup cook down a bit before adding more (creating nice, strong gravy).
6. Cover and simmer for 45 minutes, stirring occasionally. Add sugar and paprika, then salt or salt-substitute and pepper to taste.
7. Serve over wide noodles.

This low-fat recipe replaces red meat with poultry for a hearty and healthy goulash. Poultry is a good source of protein.

Turkey Burgers

MAKES 4 SERVINGS

These patties are delicious as an entrée!

- 2 *slices bread*
- 1 *medium onion, minced*
- 2 *tablespoons canola oil*
- 24 *ounces ground turkey, extra lean*
- 1 *tablespoon parsley, minced*
- 1 *egg*
- 1 *teaspoon salt or salt-substitute*
- *pepper to taste*
- 1 *tablespoon Maggi seasoning*

1. Soak bread in water for 5 minutes, then squeeze out all the water completely.
2. In large skillet, sauté onion in 1 tablespoon oil until browned, stirring frequently.
3. In large bowl, mix sautéed onion with turkey and bread, parsley, egg, salt or salt-substitute, pepper, and Maggi. Add a little water, if too dry.
4. Form palm-sized patties and fry in remaining tablespoon oil until golden brown on each side (until well done). Use a nonstick pan if possible. Drain on paper towel.

Ground turkey makes a much lighter and lower-in-fat burger than ground red meat. Be certain to choose extra-lean turkey.

Salmon Croquettes

MAKES 2 SERVINGS

This recipe is always pleasing. It's light and tastes so good!

> 2 6-ounce cans salmon, skinned and boneless
>
> juice of half a medium-sized lemon
>
> 1 tablespoon parsley, finely chopped
>
> 1 egg white
>
> 3/4 cup matzoh meal or plain bread crumbs
>
> 1 1/2 tablespoons canola oil for frying

1. Mix salmon in a medium bowl with lemon juice, parsley, egg white, and matzoh meal (or bread crumbs). If mixture is too wet, add more bread crumbs. Season to taste with salt-substitute and pepper.

2. Form flat patties, the size of your palm.

3. Heat oil in frying pan and fry patties until medium golden brown on each side.

4. Serve with a light cucumber salad or between 2 slices of crusty sourdough bread.

Salmon is one of the best sources of omega-3 fatty acids, which have recently been shown to be very beneficial to your health. This recipe is a wonderful substitute for hamburgers and makes great leftovers for sandwiches the next day.

Vegetable Chili

MAKES 6 SERVINGS

After the spices and vegetables mingle overnight, the chili is even tastier.

1 *tablespoon olive oil*

1 *large onion, finely diced*

5 *carrots, peeled and sliced*

2 *red bell peppers, cored, seeded, and diced*

3 *stalks celery, diced*

3 *cloves garlic, finely minced*

1 *teaspoon cumin*

$1^1/2$ *tablespoons chili powder*

1 *small jalapeno pepper, minced (optional)*

pepper and salt or salt-substitute to taste

1 *cup water*

1 *28-ounce can chopped tomatoes*

2 *tablespoons sherry, or $^1/4$ cup beer (optional)*

1 *15-ounce can black beans*

1 *15-ounce can red kidney beans*

nonfat plain yogurt, chopped scallions, shredded cheddar cheese (optional) for garnish

1. Coat the inside bottom of a large heavy saucepan with olive oil and heat over medium-high heat. Add onion, carrots, red bell pepper, celery, and garlic. Cook, stirring frequently, for 10 minutes, or until the onion is translucent.

2. Stir in cumin, chili powder, jalapeno, water, tomatoes, and sherry or beer. Season to taste with pepper and salt or salt-substitute. Bring to a boil.

3. Lower heat and cover. Simmer for 15 minutes.

4. Add beans, cover, and cook for 5 minutes. Uncover pan and continue cooking until the liquid has thickened slightly.

5. Top each serving with spoonful of yogurt, chopped scallions, and shredded cheese.

A good, hearty vegetable chili provides a high-energy, healthful meal. This chili contains only healthy monounsaturated fat and is loaded with fiber, protein, and vitamins. Serve this dish over brown rice, and you'll get even more fiber.

Pasta with Lentil Tomato Sauce

MAKES 4 SERVINGS

Even spaghetti and meatball lovers will rave about this dish! Lentils give this recipe great flavor and texture.

2 *teaspoons olive oil*

1 *medium carrot, thinly sliced*

1 *medium onion, diced*

3 *cloves garlic, minced*

1 *28-ounce can whole peeled tomatoes*

1 *teaspoon Italian herbs (i.e. basil, parsley, oregano)*

salt or salt-substitute, pepper, and sugar to taste

1 *cup dried brown or green lentils*

1 *pound package of spaghetti*

1. Heat olive oil in medium-sized pot and sauté carrot, onion, and garlic over medium heat for about 5 minutes. Stir frequently so garlic doesn't burn.

2. Empty the canned tomatoes together with the liquid into a medium-sized bowl and mash with potato masher.

3. Add mashed tomatoes, Italian herbs, and lentils to sautéed vegetables and stir well. Simmer over low to medium heat for about 40 minutes, adding water if it's needed to keep sauce from becoming too thick. The sauce should have the consistency of a meat or a Bolognese sauce. Season to taste with pepper, sugar, and salt or salt-substitute.

4. Cook spaghetti in boiling water al dente and mix together with sauce; serve.

Lentils are easy to prepare. They are the only legume that does not have to be presoaked before cooking.

DESSERTS

Apple Pie Nany

MAKES 6 SERVINGS

This pie is easy to prepare and tastes heavenly. It proves you can indulge in dessert without loading up on fat and calories.

$^1/_2$ *of a* 17$^1/_4$*-ounce package frozen puff pastry (Pepperidge Farm is excellent; use 1 sheet)*

3 *large apples, peeled and shredded*

2 *tablespoons honey*

2 *tablespoons raisins, rinsed with water*

3 *tablespoons walnuts or pecans, chopped and toasted*

1. Preheat oven to 400 degrees.
2. Thaw puff pastry sheet until it unfolds easily without breaking. Lay it in a 9-inch or 10-inch glass pie plate.
3. Combine apples, honey, raisins, and nuts. Spread evenly over pastry sheet.
4. Bake pie on lower oven rack for 20 minutes or until sides are just turning brown.
5. Let cool and serve.

Apple pie is an American classic, but most traditional recipes are heavy with butter and sugar. Instead of a high-fat, buttery crust, this recipe uses a light puff pastry. A bit of honey enhances the natural sweetness of apples without adding lots of sugar. For a tart variation, use raspberries instead of apples. In summertime, use fresh strawberries. This low-fat apple pie will satisfy even the sweetest tooth!

Fresh Fruit Freeze

MAKES 4 SERVINGS

Children and adults alike will love this dessert.

6 *frozen bananas (peel bananas and wrap in plastic wrap before freezing), cut into chunks*

OR

2 *cups any frozen fruit, cut into chunks*

1 *tablespoon honey (optional)*

$^1/_2$ *cup vanilla soy milk (optional)*

1. Place frozen fruit in a food processor or blender. Add honey and soy milk (if desired) and process or blend until creamy, but let some small chunks of fruit remain.
2. Transfer to bowls and serve immediately. There are many wonderful, low-fat as well as nondairy alternatives to ice cream.

Our favorite is this pure fruit dessert. It is so simple, and it's sweetened by nature. Frozen bananas make an especially creamy fruit freeze, but you can try this recipe with all of your favorite fruits—strawberries, peaches, raspberries. . . . Use your imagination! Honey and soy milk make a creamier dessert but are optional.

Enjoy eating healthfully. Be creative! We surely liked sharing some of our meals with you . . . *bon appétit!*

WEIGHT MANAGEMENT

Weight Management

You may think that a genuine interest in consumer health prompts food companies to market products that claim to reduce the risk of heart disease or cancer or help people lose weight. Think again. Many food companies are interested in one thing—the most efficient route to extra sales. The more products consumers buy and the more of them they eat, the fatter the companies' coffers. And, alas, the fatter the consumers are likely to be, as well.

—Jane Brody, Health Editor, *New York Times*

Obesity in America is a multibillion-dollar business! Big food companies gain big when you gain big. While you grow fatter consuming the products they sell, they grow richer. Dr. Gladys Block, professor of epidemiology and public health at the University of California, Berkeley, states that what is "really alarming is the major contribution of empty calories to the American diet. We know people are eating a lot of junk food, but to have almost one-third of Americans' calories coming from those categories is a shocker. It's no wonder there's an obesity epidemic in this country."

Epidemic? When we hear that word we typically think about contagious diseases, like the flu. But it perfectly describes the situation of obesity in America. According to governmental statistics, 64 percent of Americans are either overweight (33 percent) or obese (31 percent). More women than men are obese, and more men than women are overweight. What in the world is going on here?

The basic cause of obesity is clear: Weight gain results when we take in more food energy than we need to fuel our metabolism and daily activities. In other words, we're eating more food than we use up. Many things contribute to *excessive* weight gain—such as stress, genes, and junk food. Eating out frequently, consuming larger portions of food, leading a sedentary lifestyle, and shunning exercise are among the most obvious causes.

There are no magic pills for weight loss. Loads of fad diets and conflicting, so-called scientific information usually leave most dieters feeling like a Ping-Pong ball, bouncing from the latest fad diet to the next. Our weight loss strategy is simple. It's part of a lifestyle change, because **diets don't work.**

The wildly popular high-protein, low-carbohydrate diets don't lead to long-term weight loss. Even worse, they're harmful. People lose weight on these diets because their bodies get sick with a condition called ketosis (too much acid in the body). And a sick body tends to lose weight. So what we see today are lots of skinny sick bodies. In medicine, we use this type of diet—restricting carbohydrate intake—as a last-resort treatment for children and adults with severe epilepsy, when our most powerful medicines are unable to control their brain seizures.

Ketosis is abnormal. It's what causes diabetics to lapse into deadly comas. If physicians prescribe high-protein, low-carb diets as a last-ditch effort to prevent electrical brain seizures, can you imagine the potential harm for dieters *purposely* inducing ketosis by virtually the same diet? Of course, this context is missing from all of the wild marketing hype about low-carb diets.

The authors of this book know from personal experience how easy it is to gain an extra pound or two after reaching age 50. We also know that the older we get, the harder it is to lose that weight we've accumulated each year for decades. We believe that the most simple and *only* effective strategy for long-term weight loss demands true lifestyle change. As each of us approaches our seventh decade, we eagerly look forward to achieving the same results as our Mediterranean friends! We know that this lifestyle helps lower mortality rate, even in old age!

You can achieve the appropriate weight for your body type—whether you are currently overweight or underweight—if you eat a healthful diet loaded with fresh fruits, vegetables, and whole grains. Reduce or eliminate red meats from your diet and **use portion control.**

By all means, avoid unhealthy fast foods and sweet treats like desserts, cookies, candy, and sodas. Once you're over 50, eat considerably less bread, pasta, and potatoes. Don't confuse this recommendation with the no-carb diet hype! We're simply advocating a diet lower in carbs than was necessary before the age of 50. Don't cut out carbs, but cut down.

You don't have to be a fanatic about it, but eating pure, whole foods—not refined, preserved, or chemically enhanced foods is one of the best tools for triggering and sustaining weight loss. Also, drinking a full glass of water before each meal will help you lose weight. . . . Yes, just tap water is fine.

Furthermore, why does an apple a day keep the proverbial doctor away? A fresh piece of fruit is a source of natural energy to help burn excess fat. Apples are also high in fiber, which makes your stomach feel fuller and keeps it from emptying too quickly. The U.S. Department of Agriculture is actually right on with its recommendation that people should eat five to nine servings of fruits and vegetables a day.

Some Momentous Implications of Obesity

Let's be very clear about why obesity is such a major concern. Obesity contributes to the development of heart disease, hypertension, high cholesterol, type 2 diabetes, gallbladder disease, arthritis, sleep apnea, and several types of cancer. Studies show that as much as 80 percent of all heart disease and diabetes can be linked to obesity!

But there is some very encouraging news for obese people: You don't have to lose tremendous amounts of weight to significantly reduce your risk of these chronic degenerative diseases. If you are moderately obese, just losing 10 to 15 pounds or 5 to 10 percent of your weight can make a significant difference. Obese people with diabetes can often improve their glucose tolerance and the effects of insulin with only a 5 to 10 percent decrease in their body weight. However, if you are severely obese, you should get help. Start by talking to your personal physician.

It is not only that obesity is linked to a variety of chronic degenerative diseases. We believe that obesity itself is a chronic degenerative disease. As a matter of fact, it's one of the most prevalent chronic degenerative diseases of our time!

COMMON FORMS OF
CHRONIC DEGENERATIVE DISEASES

Alzheimer's Disease	Herpes Infection
Arthritis	HIV
Asthma and Emphysema	Hypertension
Atherosclerosis	IBS
Autoimmune Disease	Leukemia, Lymphoma, Hodgkin's
Cancer	Chronic Liver Disease
Cardiovascular Disease	Chronic Kidney Disease
Cataracts	Macular Degeneration
Crohn's Disease	Obesity
Chronic Fatigue Syndrome	Osteoporosis
Depression	Parkinson's Disease
Diabetes	Pulmonary Hypertension/Fibrosis
Fibromyalgia	Tuberculosis
GERD	Ulcerative Colitis

So what causes obesity to turn into a chronic degenerative disease? First of all, the fat that wraps itself around the internal organs ("visceral fat" as opposed to "subcutaneous fat," which is the stuff you can pinch on your belly) expels toxic chemicals that cause inflammation and disease, especially heart disease and diabetes. According to Dr. Richard Nesto of the Lahey Clinic, *visceral fat is a biologically active organ.* It's like a little factory in the belly that pumps out bad chemicals. This fat organ also releases fatty acids into the blood that cause inflammation and inhibit production of NO molecules. Obesity itself is a major cause of body-wide inflammation, and when fat becomes a biologically active organ it causes many other chronic degenerative diseases.

Inflammation has long been linked to asthma and arthritis, but research now links inflammation to Alzheimer's disease, autoimmune disease, cancer, diabetes, digestive disorders, hormonal imbalances, osteoporosis, Parkinson's, and heart and blood vessel disease. The C-reactive protein (CRP) blood test helps diagnose the presence of inflammation in the body, arteries, and especially in the heart. Obesity causes inflammation, which triggers an increase in C-reactive protein. C-reactive protein then chokes NO production, which in turn triggers apoptosis in the endothelium. In other words—*cellular suicide.*

But let's keep in mind the positive bottom line here: Eating healthfully and losing even 5 to 10 percent of your weight can lower the level of inflammation in your body and help you live a longer, healthier life. At this point, it should not come as any surprise to you that the Mediterranean diet lowers the level of C-reactive protein in your blood.

Obesity Can Become a Whole-Body Tumor

Obesity also has all the major characteristics of a whole-body tumor because of the virtually unlimited growth of fat cells that expand locally and infiltrate organs throughout the entire body. Fat cells can swell to as much as 10 times their minimum size and multiply from 40 billion cells in an average adult to more than 100 billion cells!

Excess fat can become a separate, identifiable part of our bodies as it coats our hearts, wraps around our windpipes, invades our livers, and spreads everywhere in the body as an organ with a life of its own, pumping out loads of toxic chemicals that cause body-wide inflammation and squelch NO production. As anyone who has tried to diet knows, the excess fat we accumulate stimulates our appetite for even more fried, greasy foods, fatty ice cream, pastries, sodas, and candy, especially chocolate. Like most slow-growing tumors, the visceral fat organ takes on a life of its own, demanding more and more "nourishment" to keep it growing.

Obesity is second *only* to cigarette smoking as the largest preventable cause of death in America. We are fast approaching the time when the number of overweight people in the developed world will outnumber starving, malnourished people the world over! Indeed, the life-threatening impact of this out-of-control visceral fat organ makes it imperative for both physicians and patients to regard it as a slow-growing tumor compromising the entire body and taking over the world's population.

You may be wondering at this point, how do you know when the amount of excess fat in the body is so excessive that it becomes like a tumor? In other words, what's the line between being overweight and being obese? First of all, take a look in the mirror. If you think you are very fat, then chances are your assessment is as good a gauge as all the insurance tables and scientific indexes. "Slightly" fat? "Moderately" fat? "Very" fat? You'll know. Between "moderately" and "very" is where the fat begins taking on a life of its own. A reasonable guideline is weighing one-third (or 33 percent) more than your ideal weight. A man who is 5 feet 10 inches should weigh about 172 pounds. If he weighs 235 pounds (33 percent more, or an extra 63 pounds), his excess fat may already be slowly growing into a whole-body tumor that will lead to further fat accumulation, diabetes, hypertension, heart disease, and associated cancers. You can be sure that your excess fat has turned a dangerous corner if you already have the Metabolic Syndrome.

The following **Body Mass Index Table** should be helpful to you.

Body Mass Index Table

Body Weight (pounds)

Height (inches) \ BMI	Normal						Overweight					Obese										Extreme Obesity													
BMI	19	20	21	22	23	24	25	26	27	28	29	30	31	32	33	34	35	36	37	38	39	40	41	42	43	44	45	46	47	48	49	50	51	52	53
59	94	99	104	109	114	119	124	128	133	138	143	148	153	158	163	168	173	178	183	188	193	198	203	208	212	217	222	227	232	237	242	247	252	257	262
60	97	102	107	112	118	123	128	133	138	143	148	153	158	163	168	174	179	184	189	194	199	204	209	215	220	225	230	235	240	245	250	255	261	266	271
61	100	106	111	116	122	127	132	137	143	148	153	158	164	169	174	180	185	190	195	201	206	211	217	222	227	232	238	243	248	254	259	264	269	275	280
62	104	109	115	120	126	131	136	142	147	153	158	164	169	175	180	186	191	196	202	207	213	218	224	229	235	240	246	251	256	262	267	273	278	284	289
63	107	113	118	124	130	135	141	146	152	158	163	169	175	180	186	191	197	203	208	214	220	225	231	237	242	248	254	259	265	270	276	282	287	293	299
64	110	116	122	128	134	140	145	151	157	163	169	174	180	186	192	197	204	209	215	221	227	232	238	244	250	256	262	267	273	279	285	291	296	302	308
65	114	120	126	132	138	144	150	156	162	168	174	180	186	192	198	204	210	216	222	228	234	240	246	252	258	264	270	276	282	288	294	300	306	312	318
66	118	124	130	136	142	148	155	161	167	173	179	186	192	198	204	210	216	223	229	235	241	247	253	260	266	272	278	284	291	297	303	309	315	322	328
67	121	127	134	140	146	153	159	166	172	178	185	191	198	204	211	217	223	230	236	242	249	255	261	268	274	280	287	293	299	306	312	319	325	331	338
68	125	131	138	144	151	158	164	171	177	184	190	197	203	210	216	223	230	236	243	249	256	262	269	276	282	289	295	302	308	315	322	328	335	341	348
69	128	135	142	149	155	162	169	176	182	189	196	203	209	216	223	230	236	243	250	257	263	270	277	284	291	297	304	311	318	324	331	338	345	351	358
70	132	139	146	153	160	167	174	181	188	195	202	209	216	222	229	236	243	250	257	264	271	278	285	292	299	306	313	320	327	334	341	348	355	362	369
71	136	143	150	157	165	172	179	186	193	200	208	215	222	229	236	243	250	257	265	272	279	286	293	301	308	315	322	329	338	343	351	358	365	372	379
72	140	147	154	162	169	177	184	191	199	206	213	221	228	235	242	250	258	265	272	279	287	294	302	309	316	324	331	338	346	353	361	368	375	383	390
73	144	151	159	166	174	182	189	197	204	212	219	227	235	242	250	257	265	272	280	288	295	302	310	318	325	333	340	348	355	363	371	378	386	393	401
74	148	155	163	171	179	186	194	202	210	218	225	233	241	249	256	264	272	280	287	295	303	311	319	326	334	342	350	358	365	373	381	389	396	404	412
75	152	160	168	176	184	192	200	208	216	224	232	240	248	256	264	272	279	287	295	303	311	319	327	335	343	351	359	367	375	383	391	399	407	415	423

Source: Adapted from *Clinical Guidelines on the Identification, Evaluation, and Treatment of Overweight and Obesity in Adults: The Evidence Report.* Chart is not accurate for children, pregnant or nursing women, very muscular people, or endurance athletes. Further research may be needed for better accuracy in people over 65 years of age.

Like other slow-growing tumors, such as thyroid and prostate cancer, which can take decades to cause problems, obesity can be eminently curable. But, in our opinion, medical science has been searching in the wrong places: Obese individuals have appetites and eating habits that are largely controlled by their excess fat, so simply insisting that they merely need more willpower is futile! Likewise, the search for appetite suppressants has not been worthwhile, because if the drug is not strong enough, then our excess fat, which becomes a separate, identifiable part of our bodies, simply commands us to eat even more food. Conversely, if the drug is strong enough, then the side effects are likely to be dangerous, as evidenced by disastrous results in people using drugs containing Phen-Fen and Ephedra.

So where should medical science be looking for an obesity treatment? We suspect a large part of the answer lies in modifying apoptosis. After all, if excess fat causes the mass suicide of healthy cells, the cells that take their place are likely to contain fat-increasing genes.

Over 300 genes have been identified as being associated with increased obesity. It's possible that they can be somehow "switched on" to cause more visceral fat in the body, which takes on a life of its own as a whole-body tumor. Dr. Jose Ordovas, the director of the Nutrition and Genomics Laboratory at Tufts University, has discovered an "obesity risk" gene. Dr. Ordovas believes that understanding more about genetic variations will help create effective treatments for obesity. He compares the situation to an electrical panel: "We know about certain switches and how to turn them on and off. But, in some people, the light doesn't come on when you turn the switch, because there are other switches upstream and downstream that we don't know about yet."

We suspect a similar situation applies to the hereditary tendency of children to become obese, because changes in genes that regulate the appetite in parents can lead to obesity in their children. In any case, there is a lot of genetic variation that determines whether our bodies store fat and become obese. But fortunately, our genes are not necessarily our destiny. Genes can be influenced by the the lifestyles we choose and various medications. We are only at the very, very beginning of our understanding, but we are confident that one of the answers is boosting levels of NO.

Harvard Medical School's Dr. Gokhan Hotamisligil succinctly writes, "If you have excess fat, even in small amounts, the body starts mounting an immune response—it's almost as if the body is perceiving excess calories as an invading organism." We agree and infer that apoptosis, which is triggered by excess fat, can lead to profound, chronic, degenerative disease, with all the characteristics of a whole-body fat cell tumor. As we explained previously, a major signal for initiating apoptosis is not enough NO. Thus, increasing NO is a very worthwhile goal, especially for people who are obese or overweight.

As empathetic physicians, we don't know whether we could have explained the concept of a whole-body tumor in a kinder, gentler manner. But, just as a heavy cigarette smoker knows there's trouble ahead, we suspect the same also holds true for seriously overweight people. Our book has become an atlas of sorts for an expanded role for NO in health and disease, especially in terms of homeostasis, entropy, and apoptosis. Among the hard realities to face is that excess fat is counterproductive to NO production, so the challenge is doing whatever it takes to lose weight before cellular damage is done. *The Wellness Solution* is a key to health and successful weight loss because it boosts endothelial health and NO. So, in that spirit, please read on.

THE SEVEN-DAY
MENU PLAN

We've shared some wonderful recipes and ideas for healthy nutrition and weight management with you in this section of the book. For folks who prefer more specific guidelines, we recommend the following seven-day menu plan. Please feel free to modify our suggestions to fit your personal tastes. Try to drink between four and eight glasses of water a day, along with eating plenty of fresh fruits and veggies, while avoiding refined sugar and saturated or trans fats. We are certain you'll be satisfied with our menu plan and experience early results that will motivate you to repeat the plan for at least another seven days.

Eating healthfully is a simple concept that can easily be put into practice without the need to agonize over counting calories, carbs, or fat grams. Never forget that it's crucial to use portion control and stop eating when you are no longer hungry. Drinking water is very helpful for portion control success and weight management, because people usually mistake thirst, especially between meals, for hunger. They could do just as well with a glass of water instead of a snack.

If you feel you must eat at least *something* between meals or after dinner and before bedtime, then we suggest a small handful of unsalted nuts (walnuts, almonds, pecans, cashews), perhaps with some raisins, or a piece of fresh fruit or some yogurt or sliced-up veggies, such as carrots or celery stalks. Remember, before you snack, have a glass of water.

It's important to point out that we did not write a "diet book." Instead, we are proud to present you with a menu that provides sensible recommendations to help you boost your NO and achieve homeostasis.

Finally, remember our motto, which is this:

Everything in moderation . . . including moderation.

So enjoy that occasional (small) chocolate brownie!

DAY 1

Breakfast:

1 Glass of Orange Juice or Juice of Your Choice (Fresh Whenever Possible)

1 Cup Oatmeal with Brown Sugar/Raisins/Cinnamon

1 Glass of Water

1 Cup of Green/Black Tea or Coffee, Hot or Cold

Lunch:

3 Ounces Tuna Salad with Lettuce and Tomato on Whole Wheat or Multigrain Bread

Apple or Your Choice of Fruit

2 Glasses of Water or 2 Cups of Green Tea, Hot or Cold

Dinner:

Green Salad with Low-Fat Dressing

4 Ounces Salmon Filet, Broiled, or Salmon Croquettes (Recipe on pg. 114)

Steamed Broccoli or Veggies of Your Choice (Fresh Whenever Possible)

Steamed Carrots

1 Glass of Water

Half Cup Non-Dairy Frozen Soy Dessert

DAY 2

Breakfast:

Whole Orange, Sliced, or Fresh Fruit of Your Choice

Cold Cereal (Low Sugar/High Fiber) with Blueberries, Banana, or Fruit of Your Choice

Soy Milk or Yogurt

1 Glass of Water

1 Cup of Green/Black Tea or Coffee, Hot or Cold

Lunch:

1 Cup Vegetable Soup

1 Slice Whole Wheat or Multigrain Bread

Garden Salad with Low-Fat Dressing

Peach or Fruit of Your Choice

2 Glasses of Water or 2 Cups of Green Tea, Hot or Cold

Dinner:

4 Ounces Skinless Chicken Breast or Asparagus Chicken (Recipe on pg. 110)

Steamed Spinach or Broccoli

1 Cup Sautéed Mushrooms or Brown Rice

1 Glass of Water

4 Ounces of Wine (Optional)

1 Slice Apple Pie or Apple Pie Nany (Recipe on pg. 118.)

DAY 3

Breakfast:

2 Slices or 1 Cup of Melon

3 Egg-Whites Omelet (Plain or with Veggies)

Toasted Bagel/Whole Wheat/Multigrain Bread with Low-Fat Cream Cheese or Butter

1 Glass of Water

1 Cup of Green/Black Tea or Coffee, Hot or Cold

Lunch:

1 Cup Vegetable or Minestrone Soup

Garden Salad with Low-Fat Dressing

2 Glasses of Water or 2 Cups of Green Tea, Hot or Cold

Dinner:

Green Salad with Olive Oil and Balsamic Vinegar

4-6 Ounces Pasta with Tomato Sauce and Veggies or Lentil Tomato Sauce (Recipe on pg. 92)

1 Glass of Water

1 Baked Apple

DAY 4

Breakfast:

Grapefruit Juice or Juice of Your Choice

Hot Cream of Wheat Cereal with Soy Milk or Yogurt

1 Glass of Water

1 Cup of Green/Black Tea or Coffee, Hot or Cold

Lunch:

Veggie Burger or Edamame (Recipes on pgs. 105, 98) on Whole Wheat
  Bread

Plum or Your Choice of Fruit

2 Glasses of Water or 2 Cups of Green Tea, Hot or Cold

Dinner:

4-6 Ounces Broiled Fish (Freshest Available; Salmon Preferable)

Steamed Broccoli

Steamed Carrots

1 Glass of Water

4 Ounces of Wine (Optional)

Half Cup Non-Dairy Frozen Soy Dessert

DAY 5

Breakfast:

Half Grapefruit

Cold Cereal (Low Sugar/High Fiber) with Blueberries, Banana, or Fruit of
Your Choice

1 Glass of Water

1 Cup of Green/Black Tea or Coffee, Hot or Cold

Lunch:

3 Ounces Sliced Turkey Breast with Lettuce and Tomato on Whole
Wheat/Multigrain Bread

Pear or Your Choice of Fruit

2 Glasses of Water or 2 Cups of Green Tea, Hot or Cold

Dinner:

4 Ounces Broiled, Skinless Chicken Breast or Chicken Goulash (Recipe
on pg. 112)

Steamed Spinach or Broccoli

1 Cup Sautéed Mushrooms or Brown Rice

1 Glass of Water

1 Cup Fruit Sorbet

DAY 6

Breakfast:

1 Cup Cubed Melon (Or Equivalent in Slices)

Oatmeal with Brown Sugar/Raisins/Cinnamon

1 Glass of Water

1 Cup of Green/Black Tea or Coffee, Hot or Cold

Lunch:

1 Cup Chicken Vegetable Soup

1 Slice Whole Wheat or Multigrain Bread

Garden Salad with Low-Fat Dressing

Apple or Your Choice of Fruit

2 Glasses of Water or 2 Cups of Green Tea, Hot or Cold

Dinner:

4 Ounces Roasted Turkey Breast or Turkey-Meatloaf (Recipe on pg. 111)

Sautéed Broccoli or Spinach

Mashed Potatoes or Sweet Potatoes

$1/2$ Cup Cranberry Sauce

1 Glass of Water

4 Ounces of Wine (Optional)

DAY 7

Breakfast:

Orange Juice or Juice of Your Choice

2 Pancakes with Blueberries/Maple Syrup (in Moderation!)

1 Glass of Water

1 Cup of Green/Black Tea or Coffee, Hot or Cold

Lunch:

1 Cup of Vegetable Soup

Garden Salad with Low-Fat Dressing

Apple or Your Choice of Fruit

2 Glasses of Water or 2 Cups of Green Tea, Hot or Cold

Dinner:

Caesar Salad with Low-Fat Dressing

4–6 Ounces Eggplant Parmesan or Eggplant Rollatini (Recipe on pg. 109)

3 Ounces Sautéed Escarole and Beans

1 Glass of Water

1 Cup Fruit Sorbet or Non-Dairy Frozen Soy Dessert

APPROPRIATE AMOUNTS OF WATER

A SCIENTIFICALLY BALANCED VITAMIN AND MINERAL NUTRITION SYSTEM

REGULAR EXERCISE

Appropriate Amounts of Water

Water plays a crucial role in keeping the endothelium healthy enough to produce NO. It's important that you drink appropriate amounts of water every single day. Be careful not to let your body get dehydrated. Drink water. . . . It's really that simple. Most people require somewhere between four to eight glasses of water a day. . . . Six is a safe compromise.

Water comprises about two-thirds of your body, so it is fundamental to your health. Feelings of thirst may actually be the body's signal that it is already dry or dehydrated. Drink water throughout the day, not just when you feel you need it.

Water is the basis of all our bodily fluids, including digestive juices, urine, lymph, perspiration, and lubrication for our joints. Water is vital to all cellular activities, especially as an essential transport mechanism to deliver essential nutrients like vitamins, minerals, proteins, fats, and carbohydrates throughout the entire body.

Let's be clear: We are talking here about your daily water requirements, not about general liquid intake. Milk, juice, and soft drinks are not substitutes for your daily water needs. Coffee, tea, or beer is definitely not an appropriate substitute because of the diuretic effect on the kidneys. Carrying around a water bottle or having one near you and drinking at regular intervals will help you obtain the recommended amount of water. Remember to try not to wait until you are thirsty.

Believe it or not, water is also necessary for your body to burn fat, especially if you are trying to lose weight. It helps keep your muscles toned and skin soft. Water also helps prevent and relieve constipation. Basically, the more water you drink, within reason, the healthier it is for you, so just remember throughout the day, *Water, water, and more water!*

A Scientifically Balanced Vitamin and Mineral Nutritional System

The importance of the role of a medically responsible nutritional system, taken over the long term, as in integral part of *The Wellness Solution* cannot be overemphasized. To review the reasons why, see Part Two of the book, which is dedicated to the subject. But always remember that there are no magic pills! In other words, even the most scientifically balanced vitamin and mineral nutritional system must be used in conjunction with *The Wellness Solution* to help you reduce your risk of disease. It is really that simple.

Regular Exercise

Few readers will need to read another book to convince them of the general health benefits of exercise. You already know it promotes health, especially cardiovascular health. What we have to tell you about the benefits of exercise goes *far* beyond these well-known facts, because exercise, as it turns out, helps improve endothelial health and NO production.

During the last five years, groundbreaking research has shed new insights on the most profound benefits of exercise. In 2000, Dr. W. R. Hambrecht and his colleagues published research in the *New England Journal of Medicine* that demonstrated a crucial link between exercise and improvement of endothelial health. Then, the journal *Circulation,* published by the American Heart Association, offered a study in 2002 showing for the very first time that daily exercise, combined with a low-fat, high-fiber diet, results in a dramatic improvement in oxidative stress, high blood pressure, and NO levels in the bloodstream—in just three weeks!

So, yes, we've known for a long time that exercise is wonderful for health. But what science has learned within the last few years about exercise and NO is truly revolutionary!

Exercise is one of the very best things you can do for your physical and mental health, because it stimulates production of NO and helps block its destruction by free radicals.

Exercise can even improve the effects of aging on our blood vessels. A European study demonstrates that blood vessels of very active older people can function just as well as younger people . . . *half their ages.*

The other good news about exercise is that you don't have to be an Olympic athlete to stimulate endothelial health and NO production. The revolutionary findings relate to those who practice just moderate exercise. Twenty minutes of brisk walking or jogging, four or five days a week, along with strength training three times a week is ideal. However, exercising aerobically three or four days a week is quite acceptable.

Even if you're physically challenged, keep moving. Make every effort to do what you can to stimulate your blood flow. Even if you need assistance from another person, seek that help. It's that important.

Anyone who exercises regularly knows that after those first days or weeks when it seems like hard work to gear up and get into your activity, suddenly it's not work anymore. Suddenly, you don't think twice about throwing on your sports shoes. The positive feelings generated by exercise—physically and mentally—have begun to take hold. These feelings are a direct result of the increased production of NO that exercise stimulates throughout your body and your brain.

You've heard of a *vicious* cycle. . . . Here's a *victorious* cycle. Exercise increases NO molecules, which stimulate positive feelings, making you want to exercise more! Exercise also increases the production of enkephalins. These small peptides have hormone-like effects on your brain to create a feeling of well-being.

Please read the previous paragraph one more time, because exercise is so crucial for our health, well-being, and weight management, yet most people, especially after they reach their 50s, avoid doing it.

Perhaps exercise is the first healthy lifestyle commitment we break because we tend to associate it with work. Choose a physical activity that you think is fun, and you can overcome this obstacle. The absolute best kind of exercise is any physical activity that makes you breathe a little bit faster, gets you a little sweaty, and fills you with a sense of accomplishment.

Another reason people give up on exercise is because they make it too hard for themselves. You don't need an expensive gym membership or a designer wardrobe. Basketball and mountain-biking are great, but they are obviously not for everyone.

There are simpler ways to get the same benefits. **You can make exercise easy.** Make a few trips up several flights of stairs at work, walk briskly, or jog to and from your car, parked a few blocks away from your work or the store you must visit. Just raking leaves or vigorously gardening can provide the physical exertion that's needed to stimulate health, wellness, and weight loss.

What could be easier than brisk walking? After all, you already learned everything about it that you needed to know when you were a child. It's probably the easiest and most versatile form of exercise there is. The possibilities for making fun out of it are endless and so are the benefits, not just for weight management, but also for lowering blood pressure, relieving chronic backache, enhancing libido, preventing constipation, and managing stress. Many people feel some of their most enjoyable and creative moments come when they are walking, because it clears the mental clutter to get ideas and solutions flowing.

The benefits of exercise simply cannot be overstated, particularly for weight loss. A study conducted at Tufts University involved men and women in their 60s who were divided into two groups: those who exercised and those who dieted. The people in the exercise group were required to burn up to 360 calories a day on a stationary bike, while the people in the diet group were required to eat 360 fewer calories a day than they normally consumed. Although both groups should have lost the same amount of weight, the researchers found that the people who exercised without dieting lost 50 percent more weight than the people who dieted without exercising. *The exercisers lost four times more fat than the dieters!*

Excuses to not exercise are plentiful, even with the best intentions: It's too cold; it's too hot; I'm too busy; I'm late; I'm tired; I'll make up for it tomorrow. It's difficult to understand why, because we generally feel so good afterward that you'd think we'd want to do even more of it!

Most people say they stop exercising because of a lack of willpower, but it's much deeper than that. What usually keeps us from keeping up with our exercise is stress. This is an unfortunate dilemma, because the more stress we have, the more exercise we need. This is why we are devoting so much of Part Four of this book to stress management!

It's too bad that it usually takes some type of a wake-up call to get going with exercise for the long haul—heart palpitations, high blood sugar, chest pains, shortness of breath, or, most often, your doctor's command: "You must lose weight." Don't kid yourself about losing weight—you must exercise—and don't wait until it may be too late for your health. Twenty minutes a day of simple aerobic exercise, three or four days a week, is wonderful for your health, your heart, your weight, and your stress level.

Aerobic exercise means that you become short of breath, but not so much that you can't talk. Just combine aerobic exercise with another 20 minutes of strength training three times a week, especially if you're in your 50s and beyond, when the signs of entropy, especially the beginning of osteoporosis, are becoming more and more obvious in your body.

Whether you practice your walking or jogging and strength-training together, or do them at separate times of the day, the combination of activities is a powerful prescription for health, energy, and weight loss. As you notice your progress, the motivation will take hold to make exercise an essential part of your daily life, as natural as getting dressed in the morning. Please, just do it. . . . Exercising is essential to your well-being!

Do only the exercises with which you are comfortable. Don't overdo it. If you're up to it, consider other types of exercise regimens such as yoga and Pilates. As we've said before, even if you are ill or physically challenged and for any reason unable to walk or lift weights as much as we have suggested, then do just as much as you can. Try to keep moving, and remember, don't make excuses. . . . It's that important!

In that spirit, we all need sensible, enjoyable, and easy exercise strategies—and what could be easier than brisk walking or jogging, outdoors or inside on a treadmill or even at the local mall if the weather is bad? Do it three to four days a week—or even better, four to five days a week—for at least 20 minutes each time, and get "a little huffy and puffy." Of course, if you are already more active than that—biking, running, or playing tennis or basketball—then keep it up! Exercise may be one of the very best things that you can do for yourself.

The following pages provide some basics on strength training. If you're thinking about skipping these pages because you think it's just about building muscles—STOP! Please, don't jump ahead, because building your strength is one of the surest ways to build NO.

Please be sure to check with your personal physician before proceeding with any of our recommended exercises.

Strength Training

If you are able to get to the gym or have some light weights at home, use these weights to keep the muscles in your body toned and strong, which is a very smart thing to do to keep yourself feeling good. Do not hesitate to work with a certified personal trainer. Most gyms have them on staff. Using a trainer is usually a good strategy, at least to begin with, because they can help provide motivation as well as instruction.

HOW TO START WITH STRENGTH TRAINING

Purchase one set of weights. Get weights that are fairly easy to lift, at least in the beginning. Here are guidelines:

> SMALL FRAME: Fair strength (most women)
> 3 pounds, 5 pounds, or 8 pounds
> LARGER FRAME: More strength (most men)
> 5 pounds, 8 pounds, or 10 pounds

- Start with what really feels like a **light** weight for you.

- Breathe properly by exhaling ... **slowly** ... while lifting weights, and inhaling while returning weights to the starting position.

- Do the exercise slowly, 15 times in perfect form, by concentrating on the involved muscles.

- If it was no challenge at all, then move up to the next heavier weight for the next set.

- If it was too heavy for you to be comfortable, move down to the lower weight.

- If it was challenging but something you were able to accomplish, then that is your weight!

- From now on, do three sets of 10 to 15 repetitions with this weight until it becomes way too easy. You may wish to purchase two heavier weights in a month or two.

Strength Training at Home

Lunges—for your buttocks, thighs, legs, and lower back

One Arm Row—for your back

Pectoral Fly—for your chest

Lateral Raise—for your upper arms

Upright Row—for your shoulders

Biceps Concentration Curl—for front of your upper arms

Triceps Extension—for back of your upper arms

Abdominal Crunches—for your abdomen

SEE THE FOLLOWING ILLUSTRATIONS FOR GUIDANCE.

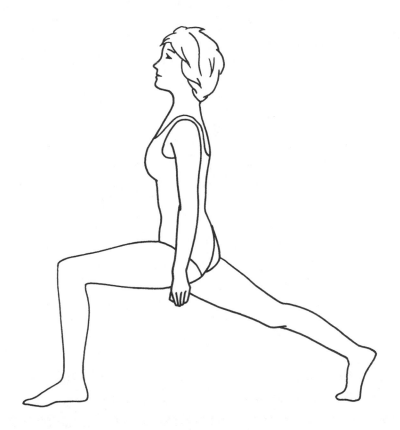

Lunges: Stand up straight with your feet slightly apart. Keep your abdominal muscles tight. Take a large step forward with your right foot. Keep your right foot flat while your left knee is pointing toward the floor. Stop for a moment and push back with your right leg, raising yourself upright again. Make sure you transfer your weight to both feet after each lunge. Do this 10 to 15 times (one set) and then repeat the exercise with your left leg. If you have any difficulty balancing, hold onto a chair by your side with one hand for support. Do two sets, taking a brief rest between sets.

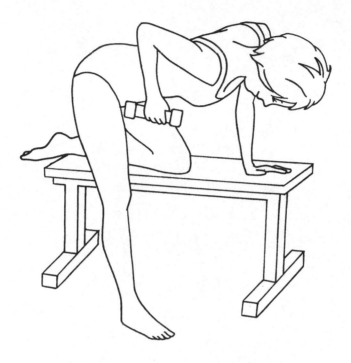

One Arm Row (With Medium Weights): Start with your right foot on the floor and your left knee on a bench or a chair. Keep your back parallel to the floor, rather than hunching up, and let your right hand hang down while holding the weight. Keep your abdominal muscles tight. Bend your right elbow and pull your upper arm as far back as it will comfortably go. Pause and slowly lower the weight. Keep the rest of your body still, moving only the arm. After you do this 10 to 15 times (one set) with one arm, repeat using your other arm. Do two or three sets, taking a brief rest between sets.

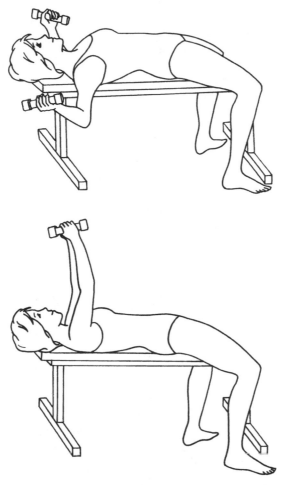

Pectoral Fly (With Medium Weights): Lie on a bench, keeping your feet flat and your hips and shoulders on the bench. If it's more comfortable, you can rest your feet with bent knees on the bench as well. Push your arms up until your elbows are almost straight with your palms facing each other. Keep your abdominal muscles tight. Pause and slowly make a wide arc with your arms as you lower them. Move your arms up and then back in a smooth arc, as if you were putting your arms around someone and then removing them. Try not to lower your arms below the level of the bench. Make sure to visualize your pectoral muscles doing all the work. Do 10 to 15 repetitions (one set) of this exercise. Do two or three sets, taking a brief rest between sets.

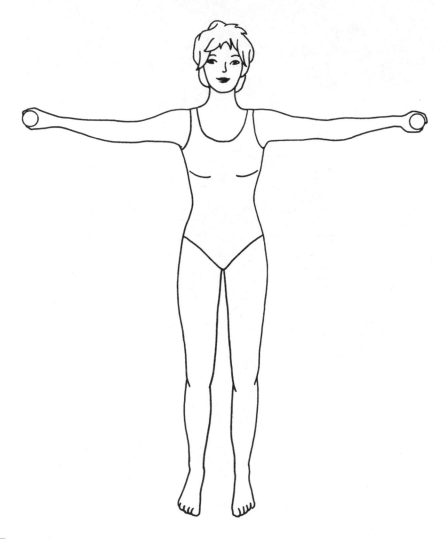

Lateral Raise (With Light or Medium Weights): Start with your feet about a foot apart, your knees slightly bent, with both hands hanging down at your sides and holding the weights. Keep your abdominal muscles tight. Now straighten (but don't lock) your elbows and lift both arms simultaneously away from your sides until they reach shoulder level. Stop and slowly lower your arms back to your sides. Don't lean forward during this exercise and make sure to keep your palms turned downward as you lift. Do 10 to 15 repetitions (one set) of this exercise. Do two or three sets, taking a brief rest between sets.

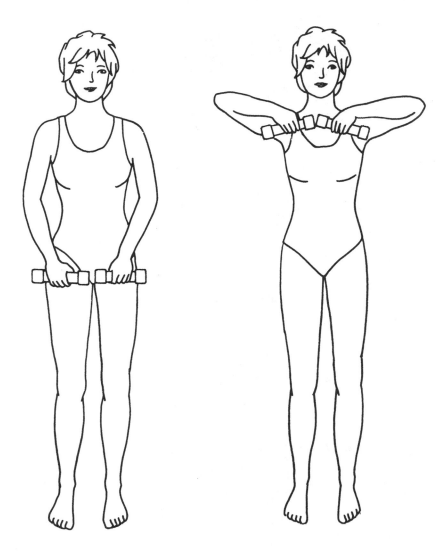

Upright Row (With Light or Medium Weights): Start with your feet about a foot apart and your knees slightly bent. Keep your abdominal muscles tight. Both hands should be holding the weights. Let them hang down in front of your thighs. Slowly lift your arms up until the weights are slightly higher than your shoulders. Stop and slowly lower the weights back down. Don't lean back or forward as you lift, and don't swing the weights around. Do 10 to 15 repetitions (one set) of this exercise. Do two or three sets, taking a brief rest between sets.

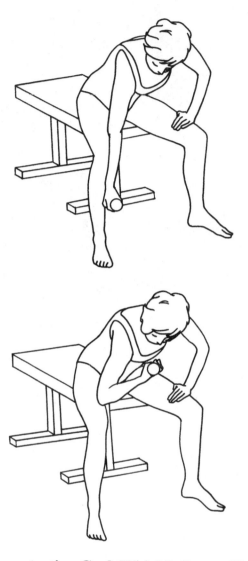

Biceps Concentration Curl (With Medium to Heavy Weights): Sit on a bench or chair with your feet more than 2 feet apart. Keep your abdominal muscles tight. With your weight in your right hand, lean forward and place your right elbow against the inside of your right knee. Slowly curl the weight toward your shoulder. Do this exercise 10 to 15 times (one set) before switching sides. Do two or three sets with each arm, taking a brief rest between sets.

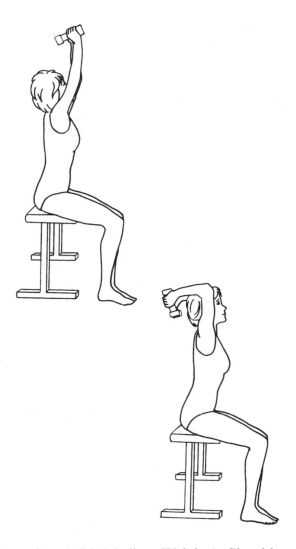

Triceps Extension (With Medium Weights): Sit with your feet flat on the floor. Push the weights up until your arms are straight. Stop and slowly bend your elbows while keeping your upper arm straight. Lower the weights until you feel a stretch in your triceps. Be careful not to stretch too far. Stop and straighten your elbows, keeping your upper arms still while slowly lifting the weights back up in an arc, so you don't hit your head. Do 10 to 15 repetitions (one set) of this exercise. Do two or three sets, taking a brief rest between sets. You may also do this one arm at a time.

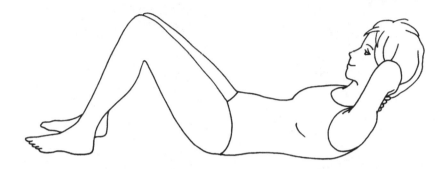

Abdominal Crunches: Keep your knees bent and feet flat on the floor. Push the small of your back into the floor. Place your hands behind your head. Use your hands only to keep your neck supported. Do not push your head to your chest with your arms. Your neck should remain in a neutral position. Raise your head, shoulders, and upper back just a few inches off the floor. Come up about 30 degrees, hold for a moment while squeezing your abdominal muscles, and then slowly lower your shoulders all the way back down. Keep going until you do three sets of 10 to 15 crunches, taking a brief rest between sets.

The Wellness Solution Exercise Plan

Do only those exercises you are comfortable with. Don't overdo it. If you're up to it, as we've said before, consider other types of exercise regimens such as yoga and Pilates. Now you can see what we mean when we say a "lifestyle change." This is the real deal to better health. Again, please remember to check with your personal physician before starting any exercise regimen. Before moving on, let's put it all together.

We consider everything we've shared with you in this section about exercise as part of *The Wellness Solution* Exercise Plan. Here's a simple summary: Completing 20 to 30 minutes of aerobic exercise, such as brisk walking or jogging, four to five days a week is ideal, along with strength-training three times a week. That is all that most people need. However, three to four days a week of aerobic exercise is quite acceptable. Of course, if you're already more active than that, keep it up.

You may substitute other forms of aerobic exercise if you wish, but make sure it gets you huffing and puffing. Remember, even if you are physically challenged, find something to do to keep moving. Finally, we recommend strength training, as previously outlined in this section of the book, because it's the only type of exercise that can slow down the muscle and bone losses that usually occur in the second half of our lives. That's it. How easy can it get?

No Smoking . . . No Excess Alcohol . . . No Substance Abuse

There is so much more to smoking than just physical addiction. That's why successful efforts to quit must include ways to overcome the deep psychological cravings behind the addiction. But take heart if you're a smoker, because over 60 million Americans have already discovered the secret to becoming a successful ex-smoker. You have to genuinely make up your mind to quit—that means failure is not an option. It requires nothing less than making a genuine commitment to yourself and to your loved ones, even promising God, if you are comfortable in doing so, to never ever smoke again.

Unless your lungs are permanently damaged by cancer or emphysema, within the very first *day* of quitting, your heart rate and blood pressure can drop to the level that is normal for your body without nicotine. Within the first *week* of quitting, your lung function and blood circulation can improve so much that your breathing and exercise tolerances are noticeably improved. Within the first *month,* coughing, sinus congestion, and shortness of breath decrease. Within the first *year,* the risk of having a heart attack decreases by over 50 percent. Finally, within just a few years, your risk of developing heart disease and cancer is nearly that of a nonsmoker.

Perhaps you've heard it said that cigarettes are the only product that when used as directed can kill you. That's because cigarettes are nicotine, tar, and carbon monoxide delivery systems that cause heart and blood vessel disease and cancer. Although most everyone knows that smoking causes cancer, most people are surprised to learn that smoking causes even more deaths from blood vessel damage and heart disease. The free radicals in tobacco smoke decrease NO levels in the blood, which causes atherosclerosis, which in turn damages the endothelial layer of our blood vessels and causes inflammation of the arteries. This is an extremely deadly, vicious cycle, because then the endothelium cannot make enough NO to replace the amounts of NO that were lost to the tobacco smoke in the first place.

Plainly put, 500,000 smokers are killed by their cigarettes every year. Smoking is the number one cause of preventable death in America (obesity, remember, is number two). Even more shocking, in our opinion, is the fact that long-term exposure to secondhand cigarette smoke, especially for spouses, children, and coworkers, is the fifth major preventable cause of death in the United States.

Smoking's effects on the body are pretty well known. Let's talk about what smoking does to your mind. Smoking enslaves your mind so much that a nicotine addict will literally say or do *anything* to find excuses to continue smoking. Sometimes smokers will even make repeated efforts to quit just to convince themselves and others, usually their spouses, kids, or doctors, that they truly want to quit. Nicotine is such a powerful drug that it causes smokers to think that they can't survive without smoking. But such nicotine-induced thoughts are far from the truth. This is why the chains of nicotine addiction can be readily broken when nicotine addicts discover the secret that once they truly make up their minds to quit, then they can do it.

The physical withdrawal symptoms from nicotine are tolerable and short-lived. *It's the mental anguish that hurts the most and lasts longest.* Nicotine itself will be out of your system in about 72 hours after your last cigarette, so any physical discomfort lasts no more than about a week. And no matter how much you smoke, the actual physical discomfort of quitting doesn't cause as much misery and discomfort as a common cold. Not too terrible a price to pay to save your life and perhaps the lives of your loved ones living with you!

The American Medical Association Strategy

Dr. Taub conducted a historic clinical demonstration among 80 patients who vowed to quit smoking for the sake of their children's health. This quit-smoking program was 95 percent successful! Inspired by Dr. Taub's success rate, the American Medical Association (AMA) used his method as the basis for its first national "How to Quit Smoking" campaign. The guiding principle behind the program's success was that participation was limited to only those patients who had first truly made up their minds to quit.

How did this uniquely effective program work? Each patient was first required to promise, in writing, to stop smoking forever and to designate a specific day to quit. Each patient also promised their loved ones and a sacred higher power in their lives that they would never smoke again. Participants basically took an oath that smoking would no longer be an option in their lives.

If you smoke, no matter how addicted you are, you can pledge to follow the same commitment adopted by the AMA in its "How to Quit Smoking" program and join the almost 4,000 American men and women who stop smoking every day, forever.

Do whatever you have to do to stop smoking. Patches, gum, inhalers, lozenges, sprays, medications, and more have helped many people. But above all, *you must genuinely make up your mind to quit,* set the date, sign a commitment, and ask someone who loves you to witness your signature. Everything else will then work out.

~ HOW TO QUIT SMOKING ~

I hereby vow on my honor and integrity,

and on all that I hold dear and sacred,

I will quit smoking forever on _____.
                                          date

_____
(Smoker's Signature)

_____
                                                    date
(Witness's Signature . . . a Loved One)

Keep in mind that you must be *genuinely* committed to quit; otherwise stress will probably be your downfall because of the myth that nicotine addicts have woven in their minds. This murderous myth is actually caused by nicotine molecules that flood nerve cells in the brain.

A nicotine addict's mind is convinced by nicotine molecules that smoking gives him or her indescribable pleasure. But that's not really the case. The brains of nicotine addicts are confused. Addicts feel dependent on nicotine only because nicotine arouses familiar feelings. However, it's not because nicotine gives them pleasure. No. Nicotine convinces the addict's brain that he or she will be miserable without it. But the actual pleasure that addicts might have received from nicotine happened long ago, at the beginning of their addiction. Eventually, nicotine addicts smoke just to not feel bad. That's a big difference from the enjoyment myth that the tobacco industry promotes!

Nicotine addiction is so grippingly powerful because it stimulates feelings and beliefs, no matter how false, which sustain its survival! We recall the pleasures smoking seemed to provide in our own lives for many decades. Years after quitting, we still occasionally wake up startled from dreams in which we've been smoking again—such is the enormous mental power of nicotine! This mental power can only be defeated by a genuine commitment to never smoke again. Never!

Don't be discouraged if you've tried to quit and failed in the past. Most ex-smokers required several attempts at quitting before they discovered the power of making up their minds. Rather than saying to themselves that they were really going to "try to stop," successful ex-smokers resolved, somewhere in their minds, that they *would stop.* In any case, it's proven that each attempt to quit smoking gets smokers that much closer to success. If saints are sinners who never gave up, ex-smokers are smokers who finally gave up!

Again, vow to quit smoking forever, set a specific date for quitting, and sign the contract that makes the promise to all that you hold dear, including, if you wish, God. You can save your life once you become aware that it's the nicotine molecules drenching your brain that are producing thoughts that say you need to smoke because it's pleasurable and hard to quit. You have the power to uproot those thoughts and weed out your addiction. Your nicotine-drenched thoughts cannot imagine how powerful you will feel once you quit. The cravings that pop up during the times your brain misses smoking will usually be gone in about 30 seconds. At first, the 30 seconds may seem like hours, but soon enough, they are just 30 quick seconds. Not much to endure for a decision that will probably save your life!

We've been very encouraging to this point but need to remind you that quitting smoking is an absolute necessity, not an option. Even one cigarette can significantly reduce NO in your body for over one hour. There is no compromise about this: You must do whatever it takes to stop. If you are still convinced that you can't quit (remember the nicotine-induced thoughts?) or that you don't want to quit, there is another secret to help solve the problem of quitting smoking, but it won't become obvious until you read the next section of the book about stress management.

A Word About Alcohol and Substance Abuse

Drinking excess amounts of alcohol or participating in other substance abuse is another serious danger. If you feel this is a problem, please seek professional help—talk to a physician, therapist, minister, or rabbi and begin attending local Alcoholics Anonymous meetings or some other support group. Alcohol and drugs can easily begin to control you rather than your controlling them, so don't wait until you hit rock bottom! Consider a rehab clinic if necessary.

Do you remember the rather simplistic anti-drug slogan of the 1980s: "Just say no"? We want to resurrect that saying here and now, with new meaning, in light of what we now know about NO. NO builds and develops the psychological and spiritual strengths that are often required to build good health.

STRESS MANAGEMENT . . . ALONG WITH BEING A GOOD PERSON

The NO Theory of Stress

Stress is a hidden killer, yet we usually tend to ignore its significance to our health. We all have said at one time or another, in reaction to a stressful moment or time, "I'm OK," when we really weren't.

NO, as an invisible gas, acts like a bridge between the body and mind. Through NO, dominant emotions are transmitted between the body and the mind. We have reason to believe that insufficient amounts of NO trigger negative messages of anger, fear, hurt, and worry, while sufficient amounts of NO transmit positive messages of resilience, hardiness, and hope. We call this the NO Theory of Stress.

Understanding the NO Theory of Stress will help you treat and manage stress in your life. In this section of the book, we lay out the basis for the NO Theory of Stress, one layer at a time, by merging the ideas of renowned neuroscientists with the molecular biology of NO. By grasping these ideas, you will have the power to put them to work to benefit your health and well-being. This is what William James, M.D. (1830–1920), widely regarded as the "Father of American Psychology," had in mind when he wrote: "Truth in our ideas means their power to work."

The only thing that can hinder the NO Theory of Stress from working for you is your already existing "stressed-out" mind-set. Thinking about lessening your stress, with the same stressed-out thoughts that created your stress in the first place, will only create more stress for you. The scientific and intuitive reasoning that follows in these pages offers you a path of clarity, a way out of a stressed mind-set, and a new understanding of the power of stress in your life and how to disarm that power once and for all.

Stripping away the stress that is affecting you is essential to successfully following *The Wellness Solution*, because with stress, you are more than likely to overlook even your most heartfelt commitments to quit smoking, drink less alcohol, eat healthfully, drink more water, take needed vitamins and minerals, lose weight, and exercise. Stress is the usual reason why people fall short in following through on their commitments.

As you learned before, NO builds the physical, psychological, and spiritual strengths required for stress management. Keep in mind the central ideas from Part One:

> *Physical* strength is necessary to slow down the chronic degenerative diseases caused by entropy—the force causing your cells to get sick.

> *Psychological* strength is needed to combat the feelings of helplessness and wanting to "give up" when keeping your healthy commitments sometimes just seems too difficult.

> *Spiritual* strength is required for you to feel worthy of making and keeping your commitments to take charge of your own destiny.

These dimensions of strength are vital to keep in mind as we now move on to explain the Simmering Stress Syndrome and its role in the NO Theory of Stress.

The Simmering Stress Syndrome

The mind is its own place, and in itself,
it can make heaven of Hell, and a hell of Heaven.
                                        —John Milton

Stress is always waging a struggle in your body. Stress can be life debilitating. It can even be lethal! Fortunately, part of the work of NO in your body, in the constant quest for homeostasis, is to prevent your stress from winning out.

Even the briefest episodes of stress that you experience in your everyday life can harm your endothelium and decrease NO levels in your body for a long time to come. It can cause your blood pressure to rise without increasing your pulse, so you may not even realize that you are stressed.

By far the most harmful and destructive stress is the stress of which you are not even aware. This is the stress that simmers silently in the background. People who are stressed out without even realizing it, especially those with inner hostility or anger, are much more likely to have heart attacks than people who realize the presence of stress in their bodies and minds.

Stress affects virtually every man, woman, and older child in America, undermining their ability to lead healthy, happy lives. Emerging research is even beginning to address the occurrence of stress in early childhood. It should not surprise us to learn that parents' stress affects their children. Infants and toddlers are wondrously perceptive and receptive, so it's only natural that they also pick up on and respond to stress in their home. Children may even perceive a parent's stressed-out behavior before the parent does! Perhaps it's because children are so busy exploring and are beginning to understand emotions. They're busy displaying their own emotions and keenly observing emotional expressions of others.

Let's look at the character and the consequences of emotional stress. We've already discussed physical stress, especially the oxidative stress caused by excess free radicals, and the chronic degenerative diseases that result. Now you should begin to recognize how deeply interconnected the physical and emotional forms of stress are.

Most readers will not be surprised by the fact that emotional stress leads to physical illness, especially chronic degenerative diseases. But the NO Theory of Stress suggests that it usually starts the other way around. *Physical stress—the state of your body—is the major cause of your negative emotions, such as fear, anger, hurt, and worry.* In other words, your physical state has tremendous impact on your emotional state.

We will talk more about the relationship between physical and emotional stress later on, but for now just ask yourself, "Have you ever come home from a grueling day at work, perhaps battling endless stop-and-go traffic, and then growled in anger at your spouse or a child, feeling your face redden, your fists clench, your jaw clench, and your heart pound, when he or she didn't really do or say anything to deserve your anger?"

Or have you ever had such a bad day with so many things going wrong that you were just plain frightened about the future and you broke down into sobs and tears? Have you ever felt your body begin to become tense, or feel short of breath, after hearing someone you care about say something or do something that was perfectly innocent?

Where do these emotional and physical reactions come from? Most of the time, it's our physical stress that first causes our emotional stress. In other words, we can become volatile, irritable, angry, hostile, frightened, or easily hurt, because the body is already physically tensed or stressed due to the bad day, week, or month that we've been having.

Let's look at this realistically. Many of us live our daily lives with a certain amount of worry. It's always there, beneath the surface, in the background, even when we stop to rest at the end of the day. This type of worry—the worry that never seems to really go away—is chronic worry. What do we chronically worry about? Most often, chronic worry is about money, jobs, the future, family problems, illness, worry about not being appreciated, and increasingly, worry about our safety in a world marked by war and terrorism. **Take a moment and write down the things that you chronically worry about.**

If money, health, and security are on your list, then you have something in common with all the other Americans who are chronically worrying about these same things. Jobs, inflation, health insurance, security—these are not just political issues. We worry chronically, because these are matters of personal well-being and happiness. Indeed, it's not going overboard to say that we are a nation of chronically worried individuals, getting by in our daily lives, but suffering at a deep level because of the enduring stress simmering away beneath the surface.

Chronic worry puts your nervous system in a constant state of alarm, so feelings of helplessness and insecurity are likely to emerge when you least expect it. So even while you're successfully taking care of things at work, at home, and in your relationships, there's that lingering sense that at any moment things might just boil over and burst! *This is the Simmering Stress Syndrome.*

Your body has its own natural stress control center—it's called the autonomic nervous system. The system is made up of *parasympathetic* nerves that generally function to calm the mind and relax the body. The system also has *sympathetic* nerves, which stimulate the production of stress hormones such as adrenaline and cortisol in our adrenal glands. These hormones keep the body and mind on the alert to respond in literally a heartbeat to problems or threats that may arise in our everyday lives. This is where the infamous "fight or flight" response originates.

Parasympathetic nerves generally function to create *calm,* while sympathetic nerves and stress hormones generally create *commotion.* The calm and the commotion that combine to create the autonomic nervous system naturally seek to balance each other. Here is the body's natural wisdom at work to achieve physical and mental homeostasis, the balance that creates peace of mind.

Unfortunately, we live amid constant reminders of worry and fear that keep our minds and bodies in a perpetual state of alert. The state of alert is even more heightened by the presence of a chronic degenerative disease in the body—because the mind becomes acutely aware that the body is suffering. Amidst this worry and fear, the body's impulse for self-preservation kicks into overdrive and lives in a state of readiness to fight or flee from perceived danger. So when do the body and mind get to relax? When do we have a chance to let down our physical and mental guards to experience the calm that is essential for a balanced, healthy life? Hardly ever, anymore.

Simmering stress is the hallmark of our time. To see this in a historical way, just look at the world today compared to the world in which your parents were raised. The differences are dramatic from the perspective of the authors' working-class experiences. Our parents worked literally around the corner from where we lived in big cities. But today's push to outsource means that jobs that were once performed around the corner are now performed across national borders. Meanwhile, tens of millions of Americans are struggling to make living wages in the face of disappearing health care and retirement benefits. While working-class families are experiencing these uncertainties, they are not alone. Middle-class and upper-class American families are also beginning to deeply feel these uncertainties undercutting the comforts and security of their daily lives.

People have always wrestled to harness the power of nature and bend its will to serve their interests and needs. Now we have powerful reminders that natural forces cannot be entirely tamed. Indeed, the body's own natural forces are struggling to restore the balance that's been lost by the demands of our modern world.

We live in a time when oxidative stress is causing widespread chronic degenerative diseases in the body. At the same time, levels of mental stress are soaring. With such a spiral of physical and psychological stress, it's no surprise that generalized anxiety disorder (GAD) has become the most common psychiatric condition in the United States. Most family doctors estimate that 80 percent of their office visits are due to GAD and stress-related illnesses. No wonder people are feeling helpless.

Take a moment to consider some of the characteristics of GAD. For many of us, some of these characteristics probably ring true to our own daily experiences.*

> ➤ Are you a worrier? Would you describe yourself as a nervous person? Do you feel tense? Experiencing a lot of worry over a six-month period is a real tip-off.

> ➤ Do you have sudden attacks of rapid heartbeat or rushes of fear, anxiety, or nervousness? Do you ever avoid important activities because you are afraid you'll have a sudden attack?

> ➤ Do you fear being watched or evaluated by others because you might embarrass yourself?

➤ Do you have any strong fears or phobias about things like height, flying, bugs, or snakes?

➤ Do you obsess? Are you bothered by intrusive, unpleasant, or horrible thoughts that repeat over and over? For example, some people have repeated thoughts that they might hurt someone they love or that a loved one has been hurt. Is anything like this troubling you?

➤ Do you have compulsions, such as doing something over and over that you can't resist, even if you try, like washing your hands very often or repeatedly checking to see that the stove is off or the door is locked? Has anything like this been a problem for you?

*Modified from Zimmerman, M. (1994). *Diagnosing DSM-IV psychiatric disorders in primary care settings: an interview guide for the non-psychiatrist physician* (Philadelphia: Psych Products Press).

Before reading further, take heart. Even if you responded positively to any of the above questions, or even if you identify personally with some of the behaviors or feelings described above, *there is good reason for you to be hopeful.*

We *can* learn how to repair the body's natural defenses against physical and mental stress—both the stress that is full-blown and the invisible, insidious stress that is part of the Simmering Stress Syndrome.

A personal example may help your understanding of stress. You probably know someone who comes from a family of brooders. When his or her feelings are hurt, or he or she is angry and upset, his or her common response is to brood . . . not just for hours, but for days. What a toll this silent, sullen brooding takes—not just on this person, but on those who live with him or her.

If you live with a brooder, you know the scenario—just as the brooder is emerging from his or her silent funk, you may be so exhausted by it that you are now heading into your own funk!

For people accustomed to brooding over the span of a few days or weeks, learning to let it go within a matter of hours is truly a monumental achievement. But hold on! New research indicates the importance of letting it go right then and there . . . literally in the very moment that the stressful emotion occurs.

It's now been discovered that the stressful situations and events in our everyday lives can depress NO levels in our bodies *for as long as four hours after* we are no longer upset. Therefore, once we are upset, if we don't immediately get back to feeling comfortable and calm before something else disturbs our bodies or emotions, then our NO levels can remain constantly depleted. In turn, the decreased levels of NO cause our autonomic nervous system, along with our stress hormones, to respond to even the most trivial or mildly upsetting events *as if they were life-threatening.* The bottom line is that our physical state causes us to become emotionally volatile, irritable, edgy, over-reactive, apprehensive, and worried. Thus, the physical state of our bodies largely determines our emotional states rather than vice versa. And the result is an enormous, constant burden on the body and mind that human beings were never meant to live with—we call this the Simmering Stress Syndrome.

It helps to recall some of the basic lessons of the "fight or flight" response. Just think about it: Emotions such as fear, sadness, anger, and loneliness can result from the way the body *feels.* Thus, people with bodies that are chronically geared up to fight or take flight are likely to be the most susceptible to constant emotional stress.

The Simmering Stress Syndrome is a relatively new condition that needs a lot more attention because the epidemic of chronic degenerative diseases and generalized anxiety disorders are reliable indicators that the usual strategies for coping with pervasive stress are not working.

The NO Theory of Stress leads to a more powerful strategy for tackling the Simmering Stress Syndrome. Fortunately, no matter what is going on around you and in you, you can still take effective steps to manage your stress. NO has the power to help your autonomic nervous system return to a state of calm and relaxation so that you can de-stress! Please read on to discover what you can do to help make this natural process happen.

It's All in Your Head

Emotional stress varies up and down with the amounts of NO in the brain and blood. In other words, the amount of emotional stress you have largely depends on NO levels in the body. Therefore, the first step you must take in managing stress is to boost the levels of NO molecules in the brain and blood. Increasing amounts of NO molecules will nurture both your mind and body. A nurtured mind and body know how to diffuse—or defuse—simmering stress.

This fact brings new meaning to this common phrase: *It's all in your head.* How many times has someone said to you, "It's all in your head"? Many people find that saying somewhat offensive or even insulting, implying that you're "just making it up." Let's be very clear that when we say, "It's all in your head," we don't mean to imply that you're making up an emotion or an illness! We really mean *it's all in your head* . . . Nitric Oxide, that is!

It appears that NO molecules transmit both your conscious thoughts and your unconscious feelings about yourself back and forth between your body and brain. To be sure, we obviously need to make a real and concerted effort to reduce and even avoid the stressors in our lives. But it's not always possible to avoid the situations or people we encounter that make us get stressed out. However, we can effectively manage stress by learning to calm the autonomic nervous system, especially settling down our stress hormone production. A calm autonomic nervous system transmits messages of wellness and security, rather than worry and fear, from the body to the brain. This is the source of an amazing biofeedback loop that then sends messages of wellness and security from your brain back to your body.

To grasp this seminal concept, you must move beyond narrow perceptions of the mind as equivalent to or just existing within the brain. You must realize that your mind is not only located in your brain, it literally exists all over your body.

Besides being responsible for the brain's capacity to think and remember, the mind is also responsible for homeostasis, entropy, and apoptosis, in every space and cell of the entire body! We've described entropy and apoptosis many times throughout this book, but the real bottom line is that they can make us older and sicker sooner rather than later. Dr. Franz Alexander, an eminent psychiatrist in the first half of the 20th century, wrote, "The fact that the mind rules the body is, in spite of its neglect by biology and medicine, the most fundamental fact which we know about the process of life."

Dr. Murad's Nobel Prize–winning discoveries opened up new possibilities for researchers to help map pathways in the brain that directly link the emotions to health. As a result, there is now a strong scientific basis, grounded in biology and medicine, for concluding that increasing NO molecules in the brain and blood is an effective strategy for stress management. The NO Theory of Stress puts these new discoveries to therapeutic use.

In science, a valid theory is a well-substantiated, logical explanation for a set of related facts or observations. Science is driven by theories—the theory of relativity, the theory of evolution, the theory of atomic structures, and so forth. Such theories are more than just educated guesses; they are the very basis of modern science. An example is the accepted fact that the world is made up of atoms: Humans, animals, birds, plants, rocks, food, and water—everything is composed of atoms, yet no one has ever seen an atom.

So it is with the NO Theory of Stress, which helps explain the fundamental dynamics in the care and treatment of stressed-out patients. The NO Theory of Stress finds its basis in several research efforts. The molecular basis of the theory comes from Dr. Murad's research. The wellness framework for the theory emerges from Dr. Taub's research. The psychological rationale is found in the research of two eminent Harvard professors, working a century apart. Dr. William James is known as the "Father of American Psychology," and Dr. Herbert Benson is the director of the Harvard Mind/Body Medical Institute.

The real value of the NO Theory of Stress is helping people realize how to help save themselves from the Simmering Stress Syndrome. Again, the idea that feelings and emotions emerge from what is going on in the body is a remarkable shift from the commonsense notion that feelings are caused by the thinking that goes on in your brain—that's the old meaning of "It's all in your head." Yet the evidence marshaled by the greatest neuroscientists of our time points to the fact that our feelings and emotions are merely a glimpse of what's happening in the body. Dr. William James's insights on this topic are especially helpful:

> Common sense says, if we lose our fortune, we are sorry and weep; if we meet a bear, we are frightened and run; if we are insulted by a rival, we are angry and strike back. My theory is that this order of sequence is incorrect. . . . We feel sorry because we cry, we feel angry because we strike back, we feel afraid because we tremble.

Just think about this. Emotions such as sadness, fear, and anger result primarily from the way the body is feeling. Thus, people with autonomic nervous systems that are chronically geared up to fight or take flight from danger are those who are most susceptible to emotional stress. In other words, you become afraid because of the way your body is already reacting.

During most of the 20th century, Dr. James's astute teachings were largely ignored in the wake of Dr. Sigmund Freud's popular theories of human behavior based on unconscious sexual tensions. Only in recent years has Freudian theory begun to loosen its grip on psychotherapy, in favor of modern approaches called cognitive therapy or relaxation therapy. These approaches substantiate Dr. James's memorable conclusion, over a hundred years ago, that the greatest discovery in the science of psychology was that human beings could alter their lives by changing their attitudes.

Cognitive therapy teaches people to substitute positive and constructive thoughts for anxiety-provoking thoughts. Relaxation therapy includes meditation, visualization, deep breathing, and yoga. Together, both therapies appear to help about 50 percent of patients with anxiety disorders. If we combine these approaches with benefits of NO and the other components of *The Wellness Solution*, we can achieve the modern antidote to stress! Again, the power of the NO Theory of Stress is its application to improve our daily lives. As Dr. James wrote, "True ideas are those that we can assimilate, validate, corroborate, and verify. False ideas are those that we cannot."

To repeat, we're talking about creating an antidote to emotional stress, especially the simmering stress of which you may not even be aware. The basis for this antidote is producing and preserving more NO molecules in your brain and blood via *The Wellness Solution*. The antidote works because NO molecules are neurotransmitters—they communicate crucial information and messages between neurons (nerve cells) in the brain and the rest of the body.

NO as a Novel Neurotransmitter

There are over 50 types of neurotransmitter molecules stored up in our neurons. These stored neurotransmitters are just waiting for the moment when the brain decides to send messages between its neurons, and eventually to nerve cells throughout the body. There are more than 100 billion neurons in the brain alone, and more messages than that are being transmitted throughout the nervous system at any given time. Imagine a busy electronics network buzzing with activity and sending signals back and forth from the brain to the body and from the body back to the brain: sit, walk, run, talk, write, sing, wash, get dressed, button your blouse, eat, cut your food, swallow, breathe, blink, pray, rest, relax, sleep, and on and on.

When neurons transmit messages to each other via the usual neurotransmitters, they do so by conveying an electrical impulse down a long, thin thread of tissue called an axon (sometimes more than a foot long) to send a signal to the neurotransmitter molecules that are stored at the end of the axon. The signal to these molecules is to jump across the gap, called a synapse, which exists between neighboring nerve cells. Aided by an exchange of sodium, potassium, and calcium atoms, the molecules eventually jump that gap, and when they get to the other side, they may or may not be accepted by the next nerve cell at the special locations called receptor sites. The neurotransmitter molecules may be rejected because there are *other* molecules already occupying the receptor sites or because the molecules don't fit into the receptor sites. Visualize the correct fit between a lock and a key. These stored-up neurotransmitter molecules generally affect the neurons in their immediate neighborhood.

Here is where it really gets interesting. NO molecules are unlike other neurotransmitters. They are unique because they are the simplest of the molecules, just two atoms that have a lifespan in the body of less than five seconds! They're also special because they are not produced in advance or stored up in our neurons. NO molecules are produced in the neurons on the spot, *at exactly the time that they are needed.* Finally, because NO is a gas, the molecules rapidly diffuse in all directions instead of having an effect on only other nearby neurons.

You can see what makes these NO molecules so amazing. There are no electrical impulses traveling down long axons, no synapses to leap across, and no unavailable receptor sites to reject the molecules!

NO molecules can move through the otherwise impenetrable cell membranes of neurons, so NO is able to transmit messages between neurons throughout the brain. In an instantaneous blast, NO sends messages to and from each part of the brain and throughout the entire nervous system to all parts of the body, including the adrenal glands, which produce stress hormones.

The movement of NO molecules forms a natural, complex biofeedback loop connecting brain and body. All parts of the body rely on NO to transmit messages back to the brain, signaling that the brain's messages have been received and either acted upon or not.

Close your eyes. Think about flexing your big toes and then do it. Neurotransmitter molecules have just been at work by transmitting the message from the front part of your brain, which is the thinking part, to the rest of your brain and then down your spinal cord and out through your spinal nerves to the progressively smaller nerves traveling down your legs, until the message reaches the flexing muscles of your big toes.

The nerve messages have just been whizzing from neuron to neuron, from your head to your toes, and because the nerves that lead to your toes also send messages back to your brain via neurotransmitter molecules, you don't even have to look at your toes to know they are flexed.

A more complex example would be moving your arm back and forth rapidly, let's say to repeatedly throw a ball to someone during a game of catch. At the order of neurons in the front of your brain, neurotransmitter molecules will relay messages to the blood vessels of your arm as well as to the muscles. The blood vessels need to relax and widen because more blood and warmth will be needed for sustained muscle movement. When you're done playing catch, the neurotransmitter molecules will alert the brain that the arm is back at your side and at rest.

Consider this final example. When a male has an erection, it occurs because the brain uses NO molecules to signal blood vessels in the pelvis to relax and deliver more blood. This is, in large part, the story behind the success of Viagra.

To sum up, it's complicated for neurons to store and release their neurotransmitter molecules with precision and speed. Neurons store up neurotransmitter molecules like torpedoes that must wait to be released by electric signals. The molecules then travel along vast numbers of long axons, jumping over the synapses between them, always seeking distant sites to land on—sites which may already be occupied by other molecules.

But NO, amazingly enough, breaks all the rules! NO gas is produced by neurons just when it's needed and transmits their messages in a flash. NO dances, if you will, to its own tune.

Mind and Body

We've all heard this question, at one time or another: Which came first . . . the chicken or the egg? We can make an argument for the egg, because without the egg, you wouldn't have the chicken. We can also make an argument for the chicken, because without the chicken, you wouldn't have the egg. So, that's the dilemma, and the answer has never surfaced. We are applying that same dilemma to this question: Is it the body-mind or mind-body connection? The following information will give you some insight into what this is all about. Make up your own mind.

Remember, the cause of psychological stress is not the troubling events and people in your life. Your stress levels reflect your mind's interpretation of what is going on throughout your body. The simplest way to understand the NO Theory of Stress is to realize that folks who have the most confidence in their ability to cope with upsetting situations are generally the folks with the lowest levels of stress. You already know how NO molecules help your body stay healthy by stimulating homeostasis, slowing down entropy, and regulating apoptosis. We can now also apply these same principles of NO to psychological stress.

Program Your Conscious Mind

You can program your conscious mind, which generally resides in the cortex in front of your brain, to think more positive, constructive thoughts. You can do this because NO molecules spread your thoughts instantaneously through the billions of neurons involved in thinking and then throughout the rest of your brain to eventually impact the autonomic nervous system via the hippocampus area near the middle of the brain and the medulla in back of the brain. This is a decisive step in effective stress management. Thoughts help determine feelings and emotions. Thoughts can communicate happiness and joy, instead of fear and worry, to the autonomic nervous system and the adrenal glands.

However, thinking positive thoughts—*Things will get better,* or *I can cope,* or *I have strength,* or *I can overlook this,* or *It is what it is*—is often easier said than done. This is especially true when you are already stressed out. Your thoughts need to be in the here and now rather than daydreaming about the past or worrying about the future. As we'll discuss in depth later, exercise, yoga, prayer, and meditation are particularly powerful ways to keep your thoughts stress free. But first, there is another fact about NO molecules that may be the most exciting news of all, especially if you are already stressed out.

Carrying out a new task, like learning to think more positive thoughts, activates the neurons scattered throughout the cerebral cortex of the brain. As you repeat the task, the connections between your neurons are strengthened, allowing nerve signals to travel along more easily. A memory circuit has been created! Research indicates NO molecules play a key role in memory because they diffuse so rapidly from one cell to another. This means that we can deepen the memory of our positive thoughts, just like grooves on an old-fashioned music record, to play back in our minds when those positive thoughts are needed most.

Finally, NO molecules can also rapidly transmit your positive thoughts beyond the front part of the brain, backward into more instinctual areas, where your unconscious mind resides. As we will explain in the following pages, the role of your unconscious mind in managing stress is essential.

Strengthen Your Unconscious Mind

The unconscious mind is largely responsible for how good you feel about yourself and your sense of self-worth. NO molecules can help strengthen those feelings of self-worth because positive thoughts that originate in the front of the brain are also rapidly transmitted throughout the brain. When NO molecules infuse the unconscious mind, they help boost self-confidence, self-worth, and in general your faith in your ability to cope. Remember, research shows that people with confidence in their ability to cope are generally people with low levels of stress.

Your attitude can create happy, joyful emotions that can lead to more powerful positive thoughts in your conscious mind, which eventually result in even higher levels of confidence in your unconscious mind. Positive thinking, meditation, prayer, and following *The Wellness Solution* are practices that help stimulate this healing process, because NO molecules diffuse instantaneously back and forth throughout the brain.

You should also know that it is the unconscious mind that determines much of your automatic moment-to-moment behavior, including sleeping, waking, lying down, sitting, standing, talking, listening, reading, washing, eating, swallowing, cutting food, and so on. Just as we don't think much about lying down in bed before going to sleep at night, or about putting one foot in front of the other to walk, or about buttoning a shirt or blouse, millions of folks don't need to think about whether they will eat more veggies, or use portion control, or exercise regularly, or take their vitamins every day—they just do it. Thus, NO molecules can strengthen your resolve to take better care of yourself. Shifts in your attitude and increased confidence can make following *The Wellness Solution* as automatic as brushing your teeth.

Stimulate Your Creative Mind

> *Like the wisdom of the body, the real and potential magnificence of the human spirit must be approached not only with wonder, but perhaps also with the awestruck attitude of Wordsworth's nun on a beauteous evening: 'Breathless with adoration.'*
>
> —Sherwin B. Nuland, M.D.

Positive thoughts and uplifting feelings about yourself can also stimulate the creative part of your brain that appears to be genetically constituted to experience a sense of spiritual awareness or connectedness. It's possible that those of our ancestors who had faith in a loving, protective higher power were better equipped than others to survive the vicissitudes of life—floods, famines, plagues, wars—and live to pass along their genes to the next generation.

According to Dr. Herbert Benson, director of the Harvard Mind/Body Medical Institute, being able to generate positive thoughts may be a classic example of the survival of the fittest over many millennia. His research also suggests that it is the buildup of NO molecules in the brain that triggers the spiritual yearnings and epiphanies that lead people to experience a sense of what we call "radical amazement."

Experiencing our connectedness to something sacred inspires our confidence and capacity to cope with stressful situations, events, and people. Such messages can be conveyed back to the autonomic nervous system and back to the conscious mind and unconscious mind, where they help build our confidence and capacity to cope. It's a fascinating example of NO molecules in action to help defuse the stress simmering in our minds and bodies. It triggers our spiritual yearnings and epiphanies. For readers with a more spiritual outlook, it is also demonstrates the Biblical wisdom which states: "As a man thinketh in his heart, so is he." (*Proverbs*)

Calm Your Autonomic Nervous System

Remember that the autonomic nervous system is the body's automatic stress-control command center. It resides mostly toward the back of your brain, in the medulla, and it has both calming and commotion-raising capabilities. The parasympathetic nervous system generally soothes and allows the body to better carry out everyday tasks by decreasing the heart rate and breathing rate, lowering blood pressure, relaxing the eyes, and aiding digestion.

In its balancing function, the sympathetic nervous system generally prepares the body for action in a flash. It does this by firing off warning messages through the nerves throughout the body while also triggering the release of stress hormones that help prepare the body to fight or take flight. In this mode, the heart beats stronger and faster to deliver oxygen and glucose to the muscles, blood pressure rises, breathing quickens, the pupils of the eyes widen to see better, the skin gets pale and cold as blood is reduced to send more to vital organs, and digestion slows down so that more energy is available to face the danger that threatens you. Blood glucose rises from the breakdown of glycogen in the liver, and serum lipids increase from stored fat in your cells. All these factors decrease NO levels.

This primitive commotion even causes hairs to stand on end, like those of a hissing cat baring its teeth, as feelings of anxiety, anger, aggression, or fear impact the brain and the body. Can you imagine the physical and emotional wear and tear this causes, especially for the blood vessels and heart? Imagine, too, how this commotion can lead to all sorts of chronic degenerative diseases, not to mention increasing one's anxiety and fear.

Of course, everyone needs an autonomic nervous system that fulfills both calming and commotion functions. What we're talking about here is living in a world that overburdens the sympathetic nervous system and creates unhealthy, even dangerous, amounts of commotion. We're talking about an autonomic nervous system out of balance, experiencing too much commotion and not enough calm.

Fortunately, neurotransmitter molecules like NO can transmit positive thoughts and an attitude of confidence throughout the brain to stimulate the calming part of the autonomic nervous system. Remember that nerve impulses are a two-way street.

Messages move from the brain to the body and from the body back to the brain, creating a marvelous biofeedback loop by NO molecules. This biofeedback loop broadcasts the message—*all is clear, the danger is over*—throughout the body and the brain, reinforcing your positive thinking and feelings of confidence.

By broadcasting this message over and over again, wellness messages drown out the danger messages and help stimulate the calming parasympathetic nervous system. When NO molecules are abundant in your brain and blood, your body transmits these positive messages with more clarity and your brain can receive them with less static and interference.

Mind-Body Medicine

I'm an old man, and I've had many troubles, most of
which never happened.

—Mark Twain

The power of NO to regulate the mind-body connection is so strong that according to Dr. Herbert Benson's research, NO molecules are largely responsible for the powerful placebo effects of most medications. Dr. Benson reviewed the research involving the placebo effect and found this astonishing fact: Placebo medication resulted in *significant improvement in over two-thirds of patients* with angina pectoris, asthma, and duodenal ulcers. Given no real medical treatment, why did these patients improve? Perhaps, as Dr. Benson suggests, the patients' positive feelings and hope for improvement stimulated the NO molecule levels that, in turn, improved the patients' conditions.

The amount of stress you experience is related to how you interpret events, not just the events in and of themselves. In and of itself, losing a job is a disappointment and presents challenges, and most people will experience job loss as stressful. However, the stress of losing a job will be far worse and have greater health consequences for someone who sees the situation as the worst thing ever, as just the latest in a long list of bad and unfair things to come his or her way. The amount of stress experienced with the loss of a job has less to do with losing the job itself, and more to do with how one interprets the loss.

For this reason, cognitive and relaxation therapies focus on identifying the negative "self-talk" and harmful attitudes that intensify your stress responses. Both approaches seek to replace this destructive self-talk with more realistic, positive, and constructive ways of thinking. NO is a powerful resource that can help you to develop the discipline necessary for effective stress management.

We all know that we should turn off the television more than we do, avoid candy and sugar-filled soda pop, exercise regularly, eat better, and make any number of lifestyle choices in favor of our health. No doubt you have heard before that stress is a hidden killer. Still, most people ignore its consequences for their health. Why not make a list of all the stressors in your life and then try to get them under control? If you can, try to eliminate the major stressors from your life. Listen to music, take long walks, calm yourself as much as you can. Take a few minutes for yourself each day to just close your eyes, practice deep breathing, and relax.

Try to build your self-esteem and self-confidence, which will help relieve some of your stress, by simply being a good person. This will help you mentally to feel good about yourself, which is a major step toward achieving and maintaining a healthy lifestyle.

Again, the real answer is boosting NO. This is why *The Wellness Solution* is such an incredible guide to a healthier you. It's an effective, lasting way to manage stress because it stimulates increased levels of NO in your blood and brain that help establish an automatic biological, psychological, and spiritual biofeedback mechanism, which signals your mind to just do what is necessary to keep you healthy and well.

Managing your stress is a must, and we encourage you to seek professional help if necessary. However, let's first discuss practical methods to harness the power of NO. And let's begin from the fact that truly the only thing we have to fear is fear itself. The NO Theory of Stress teaches that the fear we feel comes from the state of the body, and if we can get ourselves past the fear, then most everything else becomes possible. Thus, the NO Theory of Stress can help you even if you're not certain what caused your stress in the first place. It all begins by staying in the here and now and living with reality.

Staying in the "Here and Now"

Our greatest power against stress is the power to choose one thought over another. The problem is that your brain is processing hundreds of billions of bits of information at all times. Each moment, hundreds of thoughts are churning and chattering away in the background of your mind. With this ceaseless chatter, no wonder it is so difficult to harness your thoughts. And it's especially difficult if you are already stressed out.

Consider this interesting finding. Current research suggests that even schizophrenia and bipolar disorder may be related to lower levels of NO in the brain. Think for a moment: How often is it that your mind is wandering away from what's happening right now in your life and instead you are daydreaming about the past or worrying about the future or even both at the same time?

If you are like most people, your thoughts are almost always in the past or the future or moving skittishly back and forth between them instead of staying focused in the present. This is the immediate cause of stress when you are confronted with upsetting events and people. By responding to stress through the filter of past memories or future fears, you put your autonomic nervous system on high alert.

Our normal emotional responses, such as anger, worry, fear, resentment, sadness, and grief, to stressful situations are usually not about what is happening right now. Instead, they are about what has happened to us before, or what we fear is going to happen to us down the road. For example, the stress of losing a job might be compounded by anger over past losses or by fears that you will never keep, let alone find, another job. The worst enemies of the present are the sorrows of the past and the fear of the future.

The mind is generally on overload, constantly shuttling back and forth between what has been and what may be, sometimes at chaotic speed. Even at our most restful and still moments, the mind is chattering away all over the place. Have you ever noticed what you think about when you are in bed and ready to fall asleep? *I need to get gas before work in the morning. . . . The meeting this afternoon was awful. . . . I hope Mom is OK. . . . I hope the check I've been waiting for comes in tomorrow's mail. . . . I wonder what my bank balance is. . . . I should never have bought that expensive exercise bike. . . . I can't forget to stop for gas before work tomorrow. . . . Did I set the alarm?*

When your mind is in the here and now, situations remain what they are. They may be stressful, but they do not have to rattle and unnerve you. A bumper sticker caught our attention the other day: "It's five o'clock. Do you know where your mind is?"

It Is What It Is

> *The art of being wise is the art of knowing what to overlook.*
>
> —Dr. William James

In the pages that follow, we'll share with you an e-mail correspondence between Dr. Taub and a patient. The patient—we'll call him Jim—is the marketing director for a large manufacturing company. The story illustrates how fear, hurt, disappointment, anger, sadness—emotional issues that we all struggle with—can determine our responses to troubling events and people.

> *Jim:* I had a terrible situation at work that disturbed me so much that I'm not sleeping, my pulse is racing, and my palms are sweaty. Do you think I should take a sleeping pill or a tranquilizer? How about an antidepressant or a beta blocker?
>
> *Dr. Taub:* Tell me what happened.
>
> *Jim:* Another director in my company meddled in a marketing issue that has nothing to do with his division. It's totally none of his business! He tried to convince someone who reports to me about his point of view, and I think he maligned me in the process. I got angry with him and told him

I thought that what he did stinks and that he should pick another place and time for expressing his personal opinions. I'm still very angry and shaken, even though he might not have meant any harm. I know the whole episode threw me back to a time, about 10 years ago, when I lost my job because of a similar situation. . . . That was so stressful that the memory hardly ever leaves my brain. I guess I just had a reminder that we live in a very cruel world.

Dr. Taub: Stress, for whatever reason, is a reflection of not having enough Nitric Oxide in your body, especially the brain. Here's what happens: Your adrenals pump out too much adrenaline, your autonomic nervous system gets way out of kilter, and your body generates loads of free radicals. All this, which can be generated by your anger, hurt, disappointment, fear and worry, depletes the Nitric Oxide levels in your body, especially your brain.

You can help raise the Nitric Oxide levels in your system by eating more fresh fruits and veggies, exercising regularly and drinking lots of water, plus taking the vitamin formula I've recommended to you before. It also would help for you to pray, meditate, and think more positively by saying to yourself, over and over, "I Have Strength, I Have Strength, I Have Strength."

Finally, either accept the fact that "it is what it is" and just forgive the person who hurt you or made you angry, or tell him the truth about how you feel, which you already did. Sometimes it's also a good idea to preface what you say to such a person with the fact that it's the truth about your emotions, which are yours alone, rather than judgments about him. In other words, tell the truth about what you're feeling, but don't make pretensions about its being the absolute truth . . . that what he did "stinks." Someone once said that holding on to your anger is like holding on to a hot coal with the intent of throwing it at someone else. You are the one who gets burned.

All this sounds very clinical, but I assure you it's not devoid of compassion or empathy. It's what I'm always learning myself in the school of hard knocks, which is that you can't reason away your stressed-out thoughts and emotions by using the same stressed-out thoughts and emotions. You can only be proactive . . . and pump up the Nitric Oxide in your system.

A few days later, Jim wrote:

I've thought a lot about what you wrote and appreciate the thoughtful personal words you directed my way. I believe you have an inspired concept. Your "It is what it is" statement has been spinning me back to some kind of balance after really letting myself get shuffled around last week. Thanks, again.

At the beginning of this section of the book, you were asked how many times you have been told, "It's all in your head." You were then encouraged to realize that it "really is all in your head . . . Nitric Oxide, that is!" Here's the thing: We, the authors, have succumbed to stress, too—overeating, smoking, back pain, artery blockages, heart palpitations, even cancer. You might say we became experts! But we're conquering stress by taking the same simple steps we recommend to you, so please read on. NO is the answer for managing stress, and we're excited to share it with you. If you haven't yet been convinced of the importance of managing stress with NO, consider this insight from Dr. William James, a thinker so frequently quoted throughout this book: "If you believe that feeling bad or worrying long enough will change a past or future event, then you are residing on another planet with a different reality system."

Emergency Stress Treatment

Yes, no matter how you look at it, the answer is NO. The following demonstrates the power of NO in a profound and a unique way. Here is the true story of an ER (emergency room) doctor who became a patient and had to learn the answer of NO the hard way.

Thirty years after his residency in emergency medicine, Dr. Clint Thomas, a 58-year-old doctor in the emergency department of a small community hospital, felt a little light-headed and dizzy when he peeked into the waiting room. Already exhausted after a long shift, he saw that every seat in the waiting room was filled, with five or six more patients just standing around. Dr. Thomas began feeling a familiar tightness under his chin and in his chest and began talking to himself, softly enough so that no one else could hear: "God, I'm so overweight, out of shape, and stressed out. I've got to do something about it, but it's just too difficult."

He remembered how healthy he had felt only a few years ago, when he was playing tennis regularly, had normal blood pressure, and was generally happy . . . before his life savings and pension plan were wiped out in the "dot-com" bust. Again he began thinking to himself: *I drink too much, I don't exercise, I don't sleep well, I don't take vacations, I don't spend enough time with the kids, and I eat a lot of crap and always have indigestion.*

The ER admitting nurse took notice and asked, "Are you OK, Doctor Thomas?"

"Oh sure," he quickly replied. "I just need a short break. I'll be in the doctors' lounge while you get the chest pain in bed number 4 and the rectal bleeder in bed number 7 ready to examine, and please make sure the diabetic coma in room number 9 is getting her potassium. OK?"

Lying down in the lounge, Dr. Thomas felt some relief as the tightness in his chest began subsiding. He chewed three baby aspirins and reasoned to himself, thinking the same old familiar thoughts and tossing them back and forth in his mind for what felt like the millionth time: *I've got to do something, or I'm going to have a heart attack and die before I'm 60 years old.*

The chest pain stopped, and he began thinking with the same old familiar reasoning that now felt oddly comforting. *I can't diet. It's impossible. How can I stick to a diet when all I've got is candy and soda machines around me half my life?*

The familiar thoughts snowballed. *I don't have time for tennis anymore, and never in a million years am I going to be able to jog or run for an hour a few times a week . . . even if by a miracle I could set aside an hour. It's just impossible to just shut out the constant worries in my mind. . . .My concerns are too real. It's just much too difficult to live healthfully.*

All of a sudden, the tightness in his chest returned, and for the first time ever, he found himself gasping for breath because of a crushing pain unlike anything he had ever experienced before. It began under his chin and radiated down his left arm while spreading across his entire chest. Through tears, he pictured his wife and children, maybe, he thought, for the last time. He slipped into unconsciousness.

The doctor started dreaming that he was walking through a tunnel with a soft white light at its end. Very familiar arms and faces were waiting to hold and greet him, but he was interrupted by a shocking light as brilliant as a million suns and by a thundering voice. "Stand back!" someone yelled. "No change after shock number two! No blood pressure! Ventricular fib persists! OK, one last try!"

He felt the metal paddles on his chest and began clenching his fists, hunching his shoulders, trying to say the thing that was in his mind as he began turning around in the tunnel to go back home. "No, I'm going home," the doctor said to the people reaching for him. That's when he heard: "Stand back! Ready to shock one last time!"

The doctor pleaded, *God, I'll do anything to live healthy. I promise I will.* Someone then yelled, "Hold on everyone! We're getting a normal heartbeat. He's opening his eyes. This one's really got to be a miracle!"

A month later, in August 2001, during his first night back at the ER, Dr. Thomas saw a poster on the bulletin board: Emergency Stress Treatment Seminar for ER Doctors, September 13, 2001. He resolved he would attend. Of course, how did he know what was to occur on September 11, 2001?

Emergency Seminar

Fear and confusion reigned on the day of the stress seminar, which had been arranged for hundreds of ER doctors. Was America at war? Was there a danger of a nuclear attack or poison gas? What about smallpox or anthrax? No medical specialists in the country were more alarmed than ER doctors that day, nor did any of them need to be more alert and ready to serve.

As many people did that day, Dr. Edward Taub wondered how to go about "business as usual." He prepared to serve in his own way, to present the stress treatment strategy Dr. Thomas had read about. Dr. Taub readied himself to face and inform an auditorium full of ER doctors. They were the ones who would be on the medical frontlines, dealing with the uncertainties and possibilities of further attacks, further injuries, perhaps even war.

Here is the very same treatment strategy Dr. Taub gave during one of the most stressful days in world history. While the presentation was made for an audience of ER doctors, its message is presented here to all readers, regardless of profession or occupation, who seek to effectively manage personal stress.

PRESENTATION TO ER PHYSICIANS

President Franklin D. Roosevelt stirred our parents and great-grandparents during the worst depths of the Great Depression with the following words in his inaugural address: "The only thing we have to fear is fear itself."

Never have those words rung as true as in the last 48 hours since the terrible events of September 11. Our country was attacked for the first time since Pearl Harbor, and we have no idea yet what it means.

There may be more attacks with weapons of mass destruction, maybe with a nuclear weapon or biological weapons like smallpox or anthrax. It feels like the world is spinning out of control, and whatever happens, ER doctors will be working on the frontlines of medical care, as they always do.

Stress has become so pronounced in our lives that we've even invented a new term to describe it. "Stressed out" is the term many ER doctors wish they were not so familiar with.

ER doctors get stressed out because they work in a pressure-cooker environment. How can you possibly work a 12-hour shift that's usually like bedlam, then go home, rest up, and be there for your spouses and children, much less for yourselves, and then return again to work effectively during the commotion of another 12-hour shift in the ER?

I suggested canceling today's presentation so everyone could be home with their families during this stressful time. But your organization's president asked me instead to redouble my efforts with you to present a simple, no-nonsense Emergency Stress Treatment for dealing with the worst catastrophe that most of you have ever experienced.

Most people generally respond to stressful events with worry, fear, and anxiety. ER doctors are trained to stay alert and calm always, to move on from one urgent situation to the next, efficiently navigating the chaos going on around them. Just keep moving!

Unfortunately, as you get older, especially in your 50s and beyond, just moving on becomes less effective and less possible. We can no longer just assume that we can endure the stress and the pressure-cooker working conditions.

Eventually, something has got to give, if not at work, then at home or in your mind and body. This is why ER doctors need an effective Emergency Stress Treatment.

The Emergency Stress Treatment is the chance to live your life following a set of personal promises that you get to make to yourself . . . nothing more than simple guidelines to stimulate feelings of strength and calm in your mind as well as your body.

At this point in the presentation, Dr. Taub reminded the ER doctors that their patients gratefully entrust their hearts to them during the hardest moments of their lives. He urged these men and women to now put their own hearts into the personal promises that make up the Emergency Stress Treatment.

The following Emergency Stress Treatment was designed to help doctors in one of the most stressful specialties deal with one of the most stressful times in recent history. It has helped hundreds of ER doctors in profound ways, and it can help you too.

Please keep in mind that the Emergency Stress Treatment is not meant to replace medical care with your own physician. On the contrary, it should create a much more favorable environment for your own doctor's medical treatment to work.

As you are about to see, effectively managing stress begins with making a set of heartfelt promises to yourself. The promises are entirely consistent with *The Wellness Solution* principles. Obviously, they work hand in hand.

Emergency Stress Treatment Guidelines

➤ Promise to be a good person by behaving ethically and not doing anything you think may be wrong.

➤ Promise to stop smoking, to use alcohol moderately, and to not abuse chemical substances.

➤ Promise to do some form of exercise to get short of breath for at least 15 to 20 minutes, at least three to four days a week.

➤ Promise to make healthful food choices, drink appropriate amounts of water, and use portion control to manage your weight.

➤ Promise to take a daily, comprehensive vitamin and mineral supplement.

➤ Promise to love someone in your life unconditionally.

➤ Promise to forgive by adopting the philosophy that it's more important for you to have peace of mind than for your ego to be right.

➤ Promise to set aside time every day for quieting your mind.

We'll discuss all the above promises in more detail in the remaining pages of this section of the book. We'll also relate each of the promises to the NO Theory of Stress to explain their deeper purpose in effective stress management.

But first, you may be interested to know that Dr. Clint Thomas attended the seminar on September 13, 2001, and adopted the set of promises, along with hundreds of other ER doctors since then. He's alive and very well these days. His blood pressure is normal, and he no longer has chest pains. His feelings of helplessness have been replaced with feelings of happiness and reverence for life. Dr. Thomas is loved and admired by his family and thousands of patients, and he loves life more than ever.

Be a Good Person

Promise to do no wrong because being a good person is a very powerful antidote for stress. This means promising to do nothing that you even *think* might possibly be wrong. How will you know it's wrong? Most people just know, and if your mind doesn't tell you it's wrong, your body may tell you in other ways: Quick, pounding heartbeats are part of an autonomic nervous system response that tells you the body is gearing up to defend itself. The feeling is a pretty reliable inner guide to what is right and what is wrong. Being a good person cultivates self-value, personal responsibility, and reverence for life. This is the foundation for physical, mental, and spiritual wellness. Building your self-esteem in this way can provide the spark of confidence that you need to meet life's challenges—you'll feel worthy of happiness, appreciation, and love. Reintroducing the elemental principle of following the Golden Rule in your life is very powerful medicine! Feeling good about yourself, because you are really a good person, sets the stage for effective stress management.

Don't Smoke or Abuse Alcohol and Other Substances

We cover this topic thoroughly in the earlier pages of Part Four. If you smoke, just think about the fact that every cigarette you don't smoke adds about seven minutes to your life. You must stop smoking for your brain to receive the message-carrying puffs of Nitric Oxide coming to it from all over your body, saying that all is well in your body. If not, then the Simmering Stress Syndrome causes tobacco to kill you even faster. Following the rest of these promises will help you quit smoking forever. Also, if you drink alcohol, limit yourself to a glass of wine, a bottle of beer, or a cocktail not more than a few times a week. Alcohol is a depressant and can cause insomnia, especially if you are over age 50. If you drink to relieve stress, you are really just making it worse.

Exercise Regularly

As you'll recall, in the earlier pages of Part Four, we identified exercise as one of the single most important steps to managing stress. The best type of exercise for stress is something that you genuinely enjoy and that makes you breathe faster. The possibilities for making fun out of brisk walking are limitless, and so are the benefits. Walk in a beautiful place and stay aware of your surroundings—a park, a beach, or just a quiet street. Pay attention to the trees and color, even grass growing in the sidewalk cracks. Listen to music. Walk with someone you care for. Brisk walking reduces generalized anxiety by supporting endothelial health and NO production.

Eat Healthfully

Food is a source of nurture as well as nourishment. People eat for comfort and to feed anxiety, cure loneliness, and relieve disappointment. But eating junk food never solves your deeper aches. Instead, it decreases NO in your body and causes more stress. Real hunger is the body's signal that it requires more energy to carry out its work, but stressed-out people often mistake their emotional hunger for needing more food. As we pointed out earlier in Part Four, there are many compelling health reasons to follow a Mediterranean-style diet, with plenty of fruits, veggies, water, nuts, olive oil, whole grains, and fish, while avoiding red meat and junk food. Eating this way improves endothelial health and NO production. It reduces heart disease, hypertension, and cancer and helps relieve insomnia, anxiety, and depression.

Take a Daily Vitamin and Mineral Supplement

How many supplemental vitamins and minerals should you take? Which kind? What dose? This is spelled out in detail in Part Two. You should especially review our formula recommendations for avoiding and treating Generalized Hypovitaminosis, which decreases NO in the brain and blood. Remember, this syndrome is a major contributor to the chronic degenerative diseases that send constant signals to your autonomic nervous system and adrenal glands that all is not well, putting your stress hormones and your entire brain into the primitive mode of fighting or fleeing.

Be Loving

Love can shield you from stress. When you are loving or when you feel loved, you experience a sense of wholeness in your life that can heal the feelings of isolation and alienation that all of us have from time to time. In those moments of wholeness, the mind is still and the body is calm, secure, and at peace.

Promise to love someone unconditionally. If there's really no one in your life to love unconditionally, then choose a pet (and examine honestly why there is no one in your life to love unconditionally). Just remember that there are no boundaries for unconditional love— no disappointments, no disputes, no expectations, no blaming, and no resentment. If you love someone unconditionally, then you love him or her as he or she is, right now, right here. It doesn't mean that you give everything and gain nothing. Giving love can be the greatest healer of all. We suspect NO molecules carry the message of love. Perhaps NO generates love and vice versa. Maybe NO is love in its molecular form.

Be Forgiving

Wisdom is knowing what to overlook. Anyone can fight back after feeling offended, but it requires wisdom to forgive. Most people harbor hurt, anger, and disappointment, gathered up over years, somewhere deep in their bodies and minds. The autonomic nervous system seems to be the body's preferred dumping ground for all of this stored-up emotion. Just like toxic waste in a dump leaches into the soil, the air we breathe, and the water we drink, these physical and emotional toxins leach into the body's system, clogging arteries, ruining joints, gripping muscles, and clenching the heart. And all of this happens in service to the ego. Is it worth it?

The main purpose of the ego seems to be protecting your right to feel offended, so it's clearly a major stress generator. Try out the philosophy that it is more important to be happy than for your ego to be right. You'll see how powerful it is! Adopting this philosophy, you can untie the knots of past hurts and clear a path for your journey to good health and peace of mind.

Most of the things we insist we are right about are not really important. They're actually pretty trivial. Who was late? Who forgot to call? Whose turn was it to do the dishes? So we're not suggesting betraying your principles by putting on a smile instead of standing up for what you believe. We are just suggesting that your struggles may be less about principles and more about simply being right.

Everyone has certain emotional buttons that can be pushed. By overlooking potential offenses, you can disarm your ego's power to create stress and illness. Conflicts are not meaningful unless you decide to give them meaning. Then . . . ah, then! Then they are like snowballs, even like avalanches, and the more "snow" that piles up, the faster they roll and the more damage they do. Words you didn't mean to use (You're stupid . . . I hate you . . .) are seized upon by the person under attack, who makes them so meaningful that hurt or anger is unavoidable. Have you ever reached the point in an argument where it spins out of control and takes on a life of its own?

If you find that you are unable to forgive the people who, you feel, have caused you pain or hurt, take a long look at that inability. Confronting your hesitation to forgive others can be like staring the source of your stress right in the face; forgiving can free you from the chains to your past. It's been said that holding on to anger is like holding on to a hot coal with the intent of throwing it at someone else. You are the one who gets burned. Fortunately, raising the NO level in your body by following the other promises of the Emergency Stress Treatment can make forgiveness much easier, even automatic.

Quiet Your Mind

Often the most potent prescriptions are not for medication, but for a healthy dose of meditation. What does that mean? We've discussed the fact that when your thoughts are in the present, in the "here and now," then stressful events don't have to rattle and unnerve you. What triggers stress are thoughts and emotional responses to what already happened or we fear may happen in the future. Remorse, guilt, anxiety, alarm—these are thoughts and feelings pulling us back into the past or plunging us headfirst into the future. None of these emotions are tied to the present. Most people actually spend very little time in the present moment. How often will your mind drift into your memory or ahead in time as you are reading this very page? A quiet, serene mind is the key to avoiding and overcoming stress.

Your thoughts can be like the winds of a fierce storm constantly blowing your mind off course. When the winds are calm, you can experience great peace. You need techniques to quiet those mental storms, because just trying to "think positive thoughts" once the storms have begun is not enough. Your stressed-out thoughts are incapable of figuring out how to calm your stressed-out thoughts!

Meditation, prayer, and yoga help you center your mind in the present. When your mind gets dragged back into the past, meditation, yoga, and prayer can bring you back to the present. When your thoughts are lured into the future, these same practices can return you to the here and now, where you belong. In moments when your mind is not dragging in the past or running ahead in the future, the harmful emotions, feelings, attitudes, and memories that contribute to your stress can be neutralized. Meditation, prayer, and yoga are ancient practices of stopping the mental chatter and clearing away old cobwebs of thoughts, worries, and fears.

Yoga is beyond the scope of this book, but quite simply, when you practice yoga, you definitely know where your mind is. In yoga, your mind is right there in the posture, in the very muscle you are stretching, in the very breath you are taking. Many excellent books are available on yoga, and most communities have yoga classes offered by certified yoga teachers. There are also some good yoga videos and programs on television taught by renowned yoga teachers. Don't let your worries about not being flexible keep you from trying yoga! You can benefit immediately from the breathing techniques and mental calm, and the flexibility in the postures will develop over time.

Here is some truly amazing news: According to research from Yale University School of Medicine, presented during the American Heart Association's 2004 Scientific Sessions, patients practicing yoga reduced their risk of heart disease via improved endothelial function in just six weeks. The researchers reported that the improved endothelial function was most dramatic in patients who were already diagnosed with heart disease—a 70 percent improvement!

Prayer and its healing power would take volumes to delve into deeply. The power of prayer to manage stress and renew feelings of self-worth and connectedness is well documented. Could there possibly be a more powerful way to calm our fears and restore our confidence than the Twenty-Third Psalm?

> *The Lord is my shepherd; I shall not want.*
>
> *He makes me lie down in green pastures.*
>
> *He leads me beside still waters. He restores my soul.*
>
> *He guides me in straight paths for His name's sake.*
>
> *Yea, though I walk through the valley of the shadow of death,*
>
> *I will fear no evil, for Thou art with me.*

Meditation is learning to practice peace of mind. The Emergency Stress Meditation that follows is not tied to any particular religion, and it's perfectly compatible with whatever spiritual beliefs you embrace. Meditation effectively calms the autonomic nervous system by dissolving the troubling thoughts that contribute to stress. Meditation helps conquer stress by bringing your mind into the present moment, since worry and fear are only about the past and the future.

Much of the time our minds are like mountains of worries, fears, anxieties, and negative attitudes that won't budge on their own accord. We need to clear away the mental clutter that inhibits peace of mind. Meditation reaches into all the nooks and crannies of your mind, where harmful thoughts are buried, and just melts them. Remember, the worst enemies of the present are the sorrows of the past and the fears of the future. Thousands of scientific studies document the physiological effects of meditation, especially its calming effect on the autonomic nervous system. Even if you are living with chronic degenerative diseases, through meditation you can experience feeling at peace.

According to studies on meditation conducted by Dr. Herbert Benson, increased puffs of NO help us achieve a quiet meditative state. Once the mind achieves this state, then even more puffs of NO are released all over the body.

If you have never meditated before, or if the idea of meditation seems odd to you, just once try the Emergency Stress Meditation that follows. It will take only five minutes. Suspend your doubts or worries for just five minutes. For the overwhelming majority of people, five minutes of meditation will be enough to convince you of its positive effects on your feelings, mood, energy, and outlook.

Five-Minute Emergency Stress Meditation

The following Emergency Stress Meditation was taught to the ER doctors just after 9/11. It's extremely simple. All you need is a quiet, comfortable place so you won't be distracted. Wear loose clothes so you can sit up comfortably. How long you meditate is up to you, but make sure it's at least five minutes every day—even the busiest person can stick to that. Eventually your meditation time will increase as you learn to enjoy the stillness and dive deeper into the silence.

****

Close your eyes and relax your breathing. Breathe naturally by inhaling through your nose and exhaling through your mouth. Draw in feelings of calm with each breath.

Take in a long, deep breath, and as you exhale, relax the muscles of your eyes.

Take in another long, deep breath, and as you exhale, relax the muscles of your tongue.

Take in another long, deep breath, and as you exhale, relax the muscles of your neck, shoulders, arms, hands, and fingers.

Take in another deep breath, and as you exhale, relax the muscles of your chest, abdomen, and back.

Take in another deep breath, and as you exhale, relax the muscles of your thighs, calves, feet, and toes.

Continue breathing in a relaxed manner and imagine a warm, healing white light beginning in your heart and filling your entire body from the tips of your toes to the tip of your head.

Imagine the white light being created by NO molecules coursing through your body, making your thoughts become very still.

Continue breathing, and say these words silently to yourself, over and over, for as long as you wish...

I HAVE STRENGTH. . . . I HAVE STRENGTH. . . .
I HAVE STRENGTH

If you wish, you may also say these 3 words silently to yourself:

GOD LOVES ME. . . . GOD LOVES ME. . . . GOD LOVES ME.

Continue breathing, sitting quietly, with your eyes closed, feeling peace and calm in your entire body. Then very slowly open your eyes.

Conclusion: The NO Theory of Stress Redux

The Emergency Stress Treatment, including the simple meditation, ignites the natural healing processes in your body. It stimulates the production of NO, our best antidote to the Simmering Stress Syndrome.

Negative emotions—anxiety, worry, anger, guilt, hurt, and fear—cause endothelial dysfunction and a decrease in production of NO in your body. We suspect that the opposite is true as well. Increasing NO likely leads to more positive emotions—happiness, love, and hope—which will inspire resilience, hardiness, and a greater belief in our ability to cope with what life brings to us every day.

FOR YOUR REVIEW

THE WELLNESS SOLUTION

1. Healthy Nutrition

2. Weight Management

3. Appropriate Amounts of Water

4. A Scientifically Balanced Vitamin and Mineral Nutritional System

5. Regular Exercise

6. No Smoking . . . No Excess Alcohol . . . No Substance Abuse

7. Stress Management . . . Along with Being a Good Person

Reducing your risk of chronic degenerative diseases, especially cardiovascular disease, requires a comprehensive, proactive approach. Thus, ongoing consultation with your personal physician and our special guidelines to help you determine your own health destiny are integral parts of *The Wellness Solution*.

We are strongly recommending that you adapt our plan to bring more TLC—therapeutic life change—into your life. It's especially important if you feel you are vulnerable to any of the degenerative diseases brought to your attention.

Please be sure to complete your Personal Evaluation in Part Five. This can help you have a greater and renewed understanding of yourself that can change your life forever.

We end this part of the book with this thought:

> *Those who know distances out to the outermost stars*
> *are astonished when they discover the magnificent space*
> *in their own heart.*
>
> —Rilke

PERSONAL EVALUATION

PART FIVE

PERSONAL EVALUATION

The Personal Evaluation was prepared in consultation with the late Richard Friedman, Ph.D., Director of Research at the Mind/Body Medical Institute at Harvard Medical School.

The following three (3) sets of self-evaluation questions will be very helpful for you to identify areas within your nutrition, exercise, and happiness (stress) profile that will give you a better understanding of yourself. This "look in the mirror" will at least give you some food for thought.

HOW TO PROCEED

Read each statement and check it only if it applies to you. If the statement appears only partially applicable, check it if it is more correct than not. Calculate your total score for each statement you checked and write that number in the Total Score box. Scores for each question are found at the end of the set of questions, marked "Scorecard."

Please don't let your response to the statements be influenced by the Scorecard. . . . You might even want to cover up the Scorecard so that you're not influenced by it. Honest self-evaluation is a wonderful way to help yourself on your path to good health!

Nutrition

*Nutrition is the dynamic activity of eating wholesome foods that nourish the body. A nurturing diet emphasizes foods that replenish the body with vital energy instead of draining energy in the process of digestion. You will find some suggested healthful meals and recipes in **The Wellness Solution** section of this book.*

____ 1. I will go out of my way to buy the freshest produce.

____ 2. I am a "meat and potatoes" kind of person.

____ 3. I eat lots of fruits and vegetables every day.

____ 4. My usual meal is something I open with a can opener, or frozen food that I put in the microwave.

____ 5. I regularly eat fried or greasy foods.

____ 6. I drink plenty of water each day.

____ 7. I regularly eat so much food that I feel uncomfortable.

____ 8. Complex carbohydrates, fresh fruits, vegetables, beans, and whole grains make up the greater part of my diet.

____ 9. I rarely eat junk food.

____ 10. I often suffer with gas, constipation, or diarrhea.

____ 11. I prefer fresh foods to processed foods.

____ 12. I don't use much butter or gravy, and I use other heavy sauces sparingly.

____ 13. I am just about the right weight.

____ 14. I'd like to be a vegetarian.

____ 15. I drink lots of milk and regularly consume other dairy products.

____ 16. I often have indigestion, heartburn, and gallbladder or other intestinal problems.

____ 17. Cooking a nutritious, healthy meal can be great fun.

____ 18. I am very obese (more than 50 pounds overweight).

____ 19. I am moderately obese (between 25 and 50 pounds overweight).

___ 20. Fresh-squeezed fruit juice is best.

___ 21. I don't have time to make healthful meals.

___ 22. Most of the time, I skip breakfast or just eat dough-nuts, pastries, or eggs.

___ 23. I'll take the time to prepare a healthful meal just for me.

___ 24. I eat fresh vegetables as a snack.

___ 25. I am a vegetarian.

___ 26. I don't need meat to be strong and healthy.

___ 27. I gobble my food.

___ 28. My diet is mostly vegetar-ian (it includes chicken and fish, but no redmeat).

___ 29. I love salads.

___ 30. I don't eat red meat.

Total Your Score and Record It Below

NUTRITION SCORECARD							
1. +3	5. –2	9. +2	13. +3	17. +2	21. –2	25. +3	29. +3
2. –1	6. +2	10. –2	14. +1	18. –3	22. –2	26. +2	30. +3
3. +3	7. –3	11. +2	15. –1	19. –2	23. +2	27. –2	
4. –2	8. +3	12. +1	16. –2	20. +2	24. +2	28. +3	

TOTAL SCORE

Exercise

Exercise is the dynamic activity of developing balanced energy that strengthens your body and creates a sense of well-being. Exercise also revitalizes your body's storehouse of energy and inspires inner confidence. Remember, exercise is an excellent NO booster!

_____ 1. I consider myself to be in very good shape for my age.

_____ 2. I don't think I could ever get myself in better shape.

_____ 3. I engage in some form of vigorous physical activity, which makes me sweaty or breathe faster, for 20 minutes at least three times a week.

_____ 4. If I walk up a flight of stairs, I am out of breath at the top.

_____ 5. I dislike exercise and avoid it whenever I can.

_____ 6. I often climb stairs instead of taking elevators.

_____ 7. I am not a "couch potato."

_____ 8. I love walking and walk regularly.

_____ 9. I attend a health club or an exercise class.

_____ 10. I try to exercise even if I'm away from home.

_____ 11. I'm too old to start exercising.

_____ 12. I consider myself a very active person.

_____ 13. I have had hypertension, a heart attack, or a stroke, and I still do not regularly engage in any form of physical exercise.

_____ 14. Even the idea of yoga seems ridiculous to me.

_____ 15. I've tried exercise, but I can never stick with it.

_____ 16. Exercise or playing sports has always been a part of my life.

_____ 17. I feel out of sorts if I don't get my exercise.

_____ 18. When I've tried exercising, I usually overdo, and then I hurt myself.

_____ 19. I don't have time to exercise.

_____ 20. Many members of my family, and many of my friends, enjoy exercise.

_____ 21. Where I live, you can't get out to exercise.

___ 22. I don't have enough energy to exercise.

___ 23. I enjoy yoga.

___ 24. Exercise doesn't do you any good.

___ 25. My work requires a good deal of physical exertion.

___ 26. Exercise is fun for me.

___ 27. I believe that exercise is crucial for good health.

___ 28. I regularly do stretching and flexing exercises.

___ 29. My body is not very flexible.

___ 30. Exercise is very helpful to overcome stress, sadness, and depression.

Total Your Score and Record It Below

EXERCISE SCORECARD							
1. +3	5. –3	9. +3	13. –3	17. +2	21. –1	25. +2	29. –1
2. –3	6. +3	10. +3	14. –1	18. –1	22. –2	26. +3	30. +3
3. +3	7. +2	11. –3	15. –1	19. –2	23. +3	27. +3	
4. –2	8. +3	12. +3	16. +3	20. +2	24. –2	28. +3	

**TOTAL
SCORE**

Happiness (Stress)

Happiness is the enriching quality of embracing life with an open heart. Its source is inner contentment, rather than possessions. Happiness expands when you have someone to love or care for, something to hope for, and something to create. Happiness is essential for self-confidence and stress management.

____ 1. I wake up in the morning feeling excited about the coming day.

____ 2. I feel unwanted, unappreciated, and misunderstood.

____ 3. I enjoy my work.

____ 4. I have good friends with whom I enjoy spending time.

____ 5. I worry constantly.

____ 6. I am proud of my family.

____ 7. Simple things in life give me pleasure.

____ 8. I feel best when I am shopping.

____ 9. I get frequent headaches.

____ 10. I'm a genuinely happy person.

____ 11. I feel that the universe is basically unfriendly.

____ 12. A starry night is a thing of beauty.

____ 13. My possessions mean the world to me.

____ 14. I sleep very well.

____ 15. In the recent past, I have contemplated suicide.

____ 16. I feel that I am a lucky person.

____ 17. I don't fear growing older.

____ 18. I smile often and love to laugh.

____ 19. I am embarrassed by my family.

____ 20. There are so many bad things happening in the world that it's hard to be happy.

____ 21. I hug my loved ones often.

____ 22. I fret a lot about things I've done or should have done.

____ 23. My attitude is, if things are going well, then watch out.

____ 24. People come to me to be cheered up.

____ 25. I often feel angry for no reason.

___ 26. I wish I had a more honest relationship with my part-ner.

___ 27. I'd rather be happy than right.

___ 28. If I let people really know me, I wouldn't be loved.

___ 29. I'd see a glass as half full, rather than half empty.

___ 30. I feel that life is a wonder-ful adventure.

Total Your Score and Record It Below

HAPPINESS (STRESS) SCORECARD

1. +3	5. –3	9. –1	13. –1	17. +2	21. +2	25. –2	29. +2
2. –3	6. +2	10. +3	14. +2	18. +3	22. –2	26. +1	30. +3
3. +3	7. +2	11. –3	15. –3	19. –2	23. –2	27. +3	
4. +3	8. –1	12. +3	16. +1	20. –2	24. +2	28. –2	

TOTAL
SCORE

Now that you have completed the three (3) questionnaires, be sure you have added up your three (3) sets of scores *separately for each section.* Now go to the Evaluation Scale to find out where your balance is for each section to help you on your path to good health.

Evaluation Scale

Nutrition Score	Exercise Score	Happiness Score	Measure Your Balance Nutrition + Exercise + Happiness
32-40	32-40	32-40	LIFESTYLE IN BALANCE 96-120
20-32	20-32	20-32	LIFESTYLE BALANCE DISTURBED 60-96
10-20	10-20	10-20	LIFESTYLE OUT OF BALANCE 30-60
0-10	0-10	0-10	LIFESTYLE SERIOUSLY OUT OF BALANCE 0-30

We hope our self-evaluation exercise will be helpful to you in determining your own health destiny. If you find that your total score falls within the "Lifestyle in Balance" category, keep up the good work! If it showed that you fell into the "Lifestyle Balance Disturbed" section, try to make some adjustments so that you can get up to your full energy level and boost your NO. Finally, if it showed "Lifestyle Out of Balance" or "Lifestyle Seriously Out of Balance," why not do something about it? It's never too late to start.

Please keep reading on and take advantage of the tremendous amount of information disseminated throughout this book to help you understand how you can take control of your own health destiny.

PART SIX

WRAPPING UP

A Whole New Reality

The real act of discovery is not in finding new lands, but in seeing with new eyes.

—Marcel Proust

Congratulations for getting this far in the book. This final chapter will reinforce, by way of a summary and a review, what you have already read. No doubt you have encountered a lot of new information that probably was a little overwhelming. We hope you have enjoyed your journey to fully understanding wellness. What else you are about to discover is nothing less than a whole new health care reality—we call it the "NO Paradigm."

A paradigm is a framework or theory that holds information together in your mind. Your paradigms are the concepts of the world around you. They make it possible for you to function in the world as a loving, playing, working, and praying individual. Simply put, your discovery and understanding of NO will create a U-turn in your attitude and actions toward taking total responsibility for your health. Because of our current health care system, most Americans are in need of a serious U-turn in their lives. Does this sound familiar? OK, let's move on.

Shifting the way you look at yourself is a journey of discovery and transformation. By reading this book so far, and continuing to read on, you will discover a new health care paradigm that will transform your life forever. Seeing yourself in this new way will empower you to help determine your own heath destiny. That's what we call the NO Paradigm.

We are very serious about our mission and want you to enjoy all the benefits of *The Wellness Solution*. To be successful, you must discover the NO Paradigm. Once you do, your life will never be the same. Therefore, if you have not read the entire book up to this section, please don't read any further. Go back and read from the beginning. Be sure to fill out the personal evaluation questions, along with trying the Five-Minute Emergency Stress Meditation at least three times.

Let's just take a moment to review some personal yet universal changes we have all experienced. You had a very different view of the world around you as a baby than you did as a toddler. After all, you went from being totally dependent on your parents to walking, running, and maybe even saying a bold "no" to them when you were about 2 years old. You discovered your life was somewhat separated from your mother's and father's. What a discovery that was! And it didn't stop there. . . .

As a school-aged child, an adolescent, and finally an adult, you discovered many other paradigms as your mind withdrew from old habits and settled on new, more useful ones. For example, you discovered how to play and share with others. Do you remember when play and having fun were the most important things in your life?

We're sure that along the way some of your personal expectations were shattered and then replaced. Think of how your love life has changed with time. Love as a teenager, a single adult, a married adult, and a parent are expressed and felt differently. Our love cycles are the most indelible and profound components of our life. No wonder we remember them so well. All of the above are examples of paradigm shifts.

Changes in our love lives also remind us of the slow and sometimes painful process of learning from experience. Surely someone, maybe a parent or sibling or your best friend, tried to save you from your first (or second) heartache. Did other people's tales of heartache convince you to avoid a similar fate? Probably not. In love, as in so many other things, you had to discover each new relationship in your own time and in your own way.

Beyond our personal discoveries, paradigm shifts occur regularly throughout history. For example, everyone once believed the world was flat, until one day everyone knew it wasn't. Everyone knew the sun revolved around Earth, until one day everyone knew it was the other way around.

You might find this to be another interesting example of a paradigm shift: Did you know that until the early part of the 20th century, doctors didn't wash their hands before delivering babies or performing surgery? Millions of patients died from infections, especially new mothers with "childbed fever." Doctors everywhere then discovered that germs cause infections. That's why physicians and surgeons began meticulously washing their hands.

Sometimes certain things are so obvious that it just boggles the mind to think no one noticed them before. History's track record of taking action in response to significant discoveries is especially slow when it comes to replacing old health care ideas that become ridiculous (worthless bloodletting persisted till the 20th century) and tossing out entrenched health care institutions that no longer work. What an apt description of our present health care situation!

Think about it—everyone knows exercise is good for health and smoking is bad. Yet tens of millions of Americans still lead sedentary lives and continue to smoke. Most people won't behave more healthfully just because they know they should. Most often, something has to stop you in your tracks before it dawns on you.

We are totally amazed by the avalanche of new scientific information about NO that we are discovering every day. The remarkable reports streaming into medical journals have become unstoppable! As a matter of fact, the information about NO published just since we began writing this book makes us feel like young Marco in Dr. Seuss's classic story *And to Think That I Saw It on Mulberry Street.* Do you remember this wonderful story? Marco is a young boy in a pickle because his father instructs him to keep his eyes open to seeing interesting things on the way to and from school, but all Marco sees is a boring old horse and a wagon. So he begins imagining other things to report. How about a zebra pulling that wagon? How about a zebra pulling a blue and gold chariot? Or how about seeing a reindeer pulling a sled? How about an elephant carrying a rajah, who is bedecked with rubies and sitting on a gold throne? Marco exclaims, "Say! That makes a story that no one can beat, / When I say that I saw it on Mulberry Street." Marco is positively wound up with excitement by the time he bursts into his home to tell his family about what he saw.

We feel this way too, because we have a story about health care that's very exciting, and no one can beat it! Remember, this is not a product of our imagination. This story has a molecular basis. It's the NO Paradigm!

Anarchy and Chaos Under No One's Control

In 2005, just as we were discovering the NO Paradigm, Dr. George Lundberg, the former editor of the *Journal of the American Medical Association,* wrote an article directed to physicians that clarified our thinking about the urgency of this new discovery.

Dr. Lundberg described the present American health care system as "immensely complicated, often unsafe, and costly beyond belief." He declared the situation to be "anarchy and chaos under no one's control."

Dr. Lundberg concluded, "Since most health care already is self-care, why not empower consumers with good information so that they can take charge of their health? After all, it is their health!"

We, too, believe the answer is self-care and being a well-informed patient.

The present Republican Senate Majority Leader Dr. William H. Frist, who is a noted cardiovascular surgeon, agrees with that position. In 2005, Dr. Frist delivered a lecture to physicians, which was published in the prestigious *New England Journal of Medicine.* The senator envisioned the end of the present American health care system by the year 2015—as long as America's leaders make tough but wise decisions.

Dr. Frist wrote that the 21st-century health care system must ensure that patients have access to the safest and highest-quality care, regardless of how much they earn, no matter where they live, how sick they are, or the color of their skin. He explains that dignity, respect for people, and personal responsibility are critical for healing patients, along with an effective health care system. He said patients should be more responsible for preventing illness and disease with better information and increased attention to self-care. He called on the government to promote the development of better information so that patients can make informed choices. He believes the current system cannot begin to meet the needs of 21st-century America without a "true transformation."

We call this a major paradigm shift in thinking and the health care system.

According to Dr. Frist, the average premium for a health insurance policy for a typical family is over $9,000 a year—yet even in the best of circumstances, Americans receive only about 55 percent of recommended care for a variety of common conditions. He says, "It's disgraceful that almost 100,000 people die each year in U.S. hospitals because of poor care and medical errors."

We call this . . . SHOCKING!

Dr. Frist believes a whole new frontier of medicine will be opening by 2015. This will help us focus on delaying the onset of many chronic degenerative diseases. However, he also points out how difficult that can be when it takes physicians an average of 17 years to adopt widely the findings from new basic research.

We call that a challenge, because health is your most precious asset, and you shouldn't have to wait almost another decade to benefit from such a bold vision! Nor should doctors wait that long to discover the benefits of Dr. Ferid Murad's discoveries, for which he won the Nobel Prize in Medicine in 1998!

Please read on to continue discovering how the NO Paradigm affects you now and in the future. Your compliance with *The Wellness Solution* can make the year 2015 begin so much sooner for you. Wouldn't you just love to look back one day and know you've gained almost a decade of wellness? Why not? . . . You deserve it!

Paradigm Discovery

We know that compliance is the crucial, unrecognized missing piece to the challenge that Doctors Frist and Lundberg have presented to Americans. It's a proven fact that most patients will not behave in a healthier manner just because doctors give them new information or facts, even when patients hear that their lives are endangered. Smoking is the perfect example. People require much more that facts.

Good information must also be motivational and inspiring, so it literally dawns on us how important it is to do something about it. In our view, wellness is both a verb and a noun. *It insists on action.* Your new outlook on life will help you see yourself as the master of your own health destiny, not its victim.

Your journey to wellness begins at the most basic level, which is the atom. Everything is made of atoms. That includes this book, your chair, the floor, rocks, water, air, plants, and even your body. Your body has more atoms than the total number of the grains of sand on all the beaches of Earth, multiplied by millions.

As a mass of atoms, we all come from the same source and return to the same source, which is a universal storehouse of energy that initially breathes life into our atoms, making them very different from the atoms of rock. Maybe your atoms come from, and eventually return to, the energy of starlight. . . . Who knows?

When one or more atoms bind together, they form molecules. Your mass of atoms comes alive and stays alive because NO molecules provide the Spark of Life. Think of NO as a pilot light staying on until the end of your days. One day it will be time for your mass of atoms to fall apart under the persistent force of entropy. Remember, entropy is the force causing everything in nature, including your mass of atoms, to eventually fall apart.

The pilot light for a home furnace or kitchen stove lights up and stays alive with natural gas. It's always ready to ignite and deliver its heat energy through the burners whenever it's required. Your body's pilot light stays alive with NO gas. It spreads its life energy through your blood vessels, whenever and wherever it's needed. Stretched end to end, your blood vessels would reach over 100,000 miles in length. That's quite an incredible system of burners that is delivering the energy of life to your body!

Also, remember we discussed earlier that NO supports homeostasis and regulates entropy. Rather than being produced in a refinery, NO gas is produced by trillions of endothelial cells, neurons, lung cells, and white blood cells. In the NO Paradigm, your mass of atoms breaks down when NO is insufficient and entropy begins taking over. Then your pilot light goes off and life's energy leaves your body. But like a spark put to gas, there are things you can do *right now* to generate that spark—NO—throughout your body.

Are you beginning to grasp the idea that you are much more than just flesh and bones? If so, then you can grasp the fact that you are a living mass of atoms powered by NO. Your atoms are on a voyage through a human life cycle, eventually returning to the storehouse of energy where they originated. By being proactive and making the right health choices, and then complying by carrying them out, you will help make your atomic voyage as healthy and pain-free as possible by producing NO.

Let's dig a little deeper. . . . By constantly generating NO molecules, each lasting only a few seconds, your body can prevent rust, fat, and inflammation from clogging its extensive system of burners (your blood vessels). To put it in a nutshell, that's why it's possible to help determine your own health destiny far beyond what you may have known before reading this book. *Welcome to the new NO Paradigm.*

Here's how your atomic voyage works. As you've already read, NO molecules provide the Spark of Life and assure widespread delivery of life's major supporters—oxygen, water, and food molecules. Now let's go into new waters. . . . An atom of nitrogen bound to an atom of oxygen forms a Nitric Oxide molecule. An atom of oxygen bound to an atom of oxygen forms an oxygen molecule (O2). An atom of oxygen bound to two atoms of hydrogen forms a water molecule (H_2O). Six atoms of oxygen bound to six atoms of hydrogen and six atoms of carbon form a glucose molecule ($C_6H_6O_6$), which is basically what all food breaks down into in our bodies. When other atoms bond to these four basic molecules, they create complex DNA molecules that become the "stuff" of your genes, containing instructions for your cells to function throughout the entire human life cycle. This is not as complex as it might appear at first. Please keep reading.

As if all the above were not remarkable enough, consider the fact that your DNA molecules consist of your parents' DNA molecules, and their parents', and their parents', and so on. This ancestral mass of molecules in your body was given life with an initial breath of energy that bonded nitrogen to oxygen when the sperm of your father united with the egg of your mother.

Debating the origins of the universe or the force that existed before the beginning of life is far beyond the scope of this book. However, without stepping on anyone's spiritual or scientific toes, if you believe God first breathed life into your atoms, we suspect the divine breath, in molecular form, would be NO. If you believe in the theory of evolution, we suspect NO is the molecule that first infused life into the primordial mass of atoms that evolved into living organisms, and eventually human beings. If you believe in God *and* evolution, it's still NO that provides the molecular basis. In any event, your personal atomic voyage is something of extraordinary beauty, and the NO Paradigm helps you understand what the poet William Blake meant about seeing the entire world in a grain of sand and heaven in a wild flower.

The NO Paradigm comes just in time, especially for people over 50 who are trying to navigate the murky waters of information about chronic degenerative diseases, especially heart and blood vessel disease. Just for a moment, forget about the huge amount of confusing information "out there," and instead contemplate the information that's right before you. Your genes contain coded instructions for your cells to produce NO, which enters your bloodstream as a vital signaling molecule for health. By controlling your blood flow, NO preserves all your bodily functions. NO is virtually EVERYTHING when it comes to your health and healing. It's the total molecular basis of wellness.

NO lights up the courtship flame of the male firefly—which is seen from afar by the female fireflies determined to pass on their DNA to the future. That's just one amazing example of all the new information being released about NO's part in our lives.

Scientists have recently discovered that NO helps light up the Northern Lights and helps create the reddish glow in the nighttime sky of Mars and Venus! That's especially startling, because wherever NO exists, there is a chance of life elsewhere in the universe.

Here are some more examples of how we can boost NO to make our bodies feel good: yoga . . . massage . . . acupuncture . . . listening to calming music . . . even humming to ourselves. If that list wasn't enough to motivate and inspire you to take steps to produce more NO, scientists recently discovered that laughter—especially good belly laughs—is good medicine because it, too, stimulates the production of NO. Wow! Much to our delight, we also learned that Dr. Norman Hollenberg, a Harvard Medical School researcher and former editor of the *New England Journal of Medicine*, has demonstrated that eating high-quality dark chocolate (in moderation!) may increase NO and possibly lower blood pressure to reduce the risk of strokes. Now that's a discovery to sink your teeth into!

Finally, remarkable studies have been conducted by Dr. Robert Vogel, a preventive medicine cardiologist. His research demonstrated that smoking just one cigarette wipes out much of the NO in the body for more than an hour, and that a typical greasy, fast-food meal wipes out much of the NO for up to two hours. On the positive side, we also learned about several new studies which show that exercising regularly and eating abundant amounts of fruits and veggies are excellent ways of stimulating NO.

What finally propelled us feet first into the world of the NO Paradigm was amazing new information about inflammation published in 2005. Please read on.

Inflammation Nation

Medical science is on the verge of its own revolution in understanding the causes of chronic degenerative diseases, especially heart disease. Scientists now believe that inflammation is the major underlying physical problem. This really comes as no big surprise, considering the ways Americans eat, their sedentary lives, and the high levels of the Simmering Stress Syndrome. But remember, *The Wellness Solution* is the way for you to combat all of the above . . . and more!

Basically, here's what you need to know about the latest discoveries. Decreased NO production triggers chronic inflammation, which in turn further inhibits NO production. That's an especially destructive and vicious cycle, because producing more NO is the best response to inflammation.

It's important to understand that inflammation is your body's natural healing response to an injury, an infection, or a threat. In this light, inflammation is meant to be a good thing that protects your body and promotes healing.

Please do a simple experiment. Slap the underside of your forearm sharply. You'll see redness and swelling, and you'll feel heat and pain. These are signs of inflammation that indicate the body is sending more blood and healing molecules to your injury. If you have an infection, then the redness, swelling, heat, and pain would be part of the body's effort to isolate the germs by forming a boil. The problem, these days, is the constant injury or threat from excess free-radical molecules in all parts of the body. Remember, we call this oxidative stress—or, if you prefer, rust.

Let's look more deeply at the underlying issue of inflammation. How do we measure inflammation in the body? Measuring inflammation in the arteries is not as straightforward as measuring inflammation of the skin, which we can easily see. One of the ways we diagnose inflammation, especially in the coronary arteries nourishing the heart, is through measuring C-reactive protein (CRP) in the blood. A high level of CRP is a reliable measure of inflammation in the body. Amazingly, researchers have shown that CRP is as important as cholesterol in diagnosing and treating heart disease!

Two studies published in the *New England Journal of Medicine* demonstrated that reducing high CRP levels slows down the progression of atherosclerosis and prevents heart attacks and heart-related deaths. This was the first direct scientific evidence that reducing inflammation is as important as reducing cholesterol for a healthy heart. Believe it or not, that amazing finding was just identified and reported in the medical journals in the year 2005!

This is news that should make us all take heart! Did you know that half of all people who suffer heart attacks have *perfectly normal* cholesterol levels? It's true! So this means that by focusing entirely on cholesterol levels, physicians and patients have been missing a crucial element in addressing heart health. In other words, just fixing high cholesterol levels alone is not enough—we've got to lower inflammation levels as well. Remember, ***The Wellness Solution*** is a highly effective way of boosting NO.

It's no wonder Dr. Steven Nissen of the Cleveland Clinic, an author of the one of the studies, commented, "All of a sudden, we have a revolution. . . . We need to attack CRP with the same aggressiveness that we have used for cholesterol."

No kidding!

The above information demonstrated that cholesterol-lowering statin drugs, *the most widely used drugs in the world,* help prevent heart attacks by lowering cholesterol and lowering CRP. Now, that's both a good and bad thing. It's good, because now doctors know the greatest reduction in heart disease comes from lowering both cholesterol and CRP. It's bad, because experts are already declaring that the best hope for heart patients is taking more statin drugs! One expert has declared: "The first and most important thing to do in light of the newly published information is to increase the dosage of statin drugs to about twice the normally prescribed dose if necessary to lower CRP."

No, we disagree! This is a very good time to remind you again about *The Wellness Solution*. The first and most important thing to do is to increase NO production. It's a well-known fact that increased doses of statins are associated with a significant risk of liver and muscle damage, so we suggest to both doctors and patients that they exercise serious caution. We expect newly published research to accelerate the search for other drugs that can reduce inflammation with fewer negative side effects. In the meantime pharmaceutical firms are investing hundreds of millions of dollars to add NO-boosting molecules to already existing cardiovascular and anti-inflammatory drugs. It's also possible that the heart-health benefits of taking low doses of daily aspirin may be partially due to its positive effects on inflammation in the blood vessels.

Bi-Dil is a new drug that boosts NO. It was approved by the FDA in 2005, specifically for heart failure in African Americans. It's been discovered that African Americans are considerably more susceptible to NO deficiency and endothelial dysfunction than Caucasians. Bi-Dil boosts NO production and also acts as an antioxidant to preserve NO. The drug has been shown to reduce deaths from heart failure in sick African American patients by 43 percent. . . . This is a spectacular improvement!

While there is still a lot for the researchers to determine, right now the most important thing that you can do to reduce inflammation in your body is to wholeheartedly comply with *The Wellness Solution*. Since CRP levels can be lowered by lifestyle changes, why not start with more self-care before more drugs?

Here's another example of how important it is to reduce your CRP. In 2002, which seems like a very long time ago, given the recent flood of NO-related research, Dr. Subodh Verma and his colleagues demonstrated that increased CRP levels can directly quench the production of NO. Therefore, they wondered if decreasing CRP levels might directly reduce many diseases by improving the production of NO. Indeed, this seems to be the case with the statin drugs, which is why they are now being considered for wider usage in many chronic degenerative diseases, including Alzheimer's disease, arthritis, cancer, and multiple sclerosis. Before everyone is routinely advised to take statins, we strongly recommend complying with *The Wellness Solution*.

We are certainly *not* suggesting that judicious increases in statin dosages for patients who are at high risk of cardiovascular diseases is wrong, especially since we now know that statin drugs improve endothelial function, increase NO production, and decrease inflammation. Instead, we are pointing out what should be clear to you by now, which is that in the NO Paradigm, your health is primarily determined by your own personal responsibility, self-value, and reverence for life . . . along with the best that modern medicine has to offer. It's really that simple, and that's why we recommend *The Wellness Solution* so strongly.

Let's review some basics. Atherosclerosis, which leads to coronary artery disease and strokes, begins early in life. It results from an accumulation of cholesterol plaque in the coronary arteries supplying blood to the heart muscles. Eventually this plaque reduces blood flow, forces the heart to work harder and, if the artery is completely blocked, then a heart attack may result. Right? Well, not exactly.

Not long ago, cardiologists thought a heart attack was simply a buildup of cholesterol, eventually causing a blockage in an artery. But we know now, more accurately, that inflammation inside the blood vessels and arteries, rather than cholesterol, initially causes the plaque. Inflammation also causes the plaque to rupture and break off into smaller pieces that lodge downstream in the narrower parts of the blood vessels, where it can cause life-threatening events.

So, in summary, the story of coronary artery disease begins well before cholesterol buildup. It begins when free-radical molecules and decreased NO levels cause injury to the delicate endothelial cells lining our blood vessel walls. Remember, injury leads to inflammation. That's why cardiologists are now beginning to see inflammation as the culprit leading to deposits and build-up of cholesterol on our blood vessels' walls. The current scientific understanding of atherosclerosis, which is based on the notion that the cholesterol we ingest somehow deposits itself on the walls of our blood vessels, is way too simplistic. After all, the human body, which is such a remarkable living system of atoms and molecules, isn't so poorly constructed that it would just deposit excess fat on the inner linings of the very blood vessels that support life by nourishing its brain and heart!

It's the steady production of NO that keeps all the blood vessels, including your arteries, open and in good shape. Normal soft and elastic blood vessels help keep blood flowing smoothly to and from the heart and brain, and everywhere else in the body. Think of a healthy endothelial lining as being nonsticky like Teflon. Now imagine the endothelial lining of your blood vessels being injured because of oxidation, or rust. NO production decreases when the endothelium is unhealthy or sick. We now know that NO also helps prevent oxidation of the endothelium in the first place, so as NO levels decrease, the endothelium becomes more dysfunctional. This is a very simple way to understand how heart and blood vessel disease develops. It begins and ends with NO.

Furthermore, NO helps to keep white blood cells and platelets from sticking to blood vessel walls and forming clots. Finally, NO suppresses the accumulation of cholesterol plaque on blood vessel walls and can even melt away plaque that already exists, just like a Teflon effect . . . incredible!

Inflammation occurs because the delicate endothelial lining becomes injured when NO levels are too low. The Teflon factor rapidly deteriorates, which allows fat to begin sticking to the inflamed surface. This triggers the release of white blood cells that rush to wall off the inflamed areas, just as if it were an infection. The rush of white blood cells causes pus, mucous, redness, swelling, heat, and pain—which just results in more inflammation!

When the acute inflammation is over, the cholesterol accumulation becomes dry, thick, and less elastic, and it converts into plaque. When cracks begin forming in the hardened cholesterol, even more inflammation occurs. This is merely the body's attempt to hold the plaque together. More havoc occurs when platelets rush to the inflamed area and gather around the cracks, sticking to them in order to help them hold together. Platelets perform this task by forming clots, which make the unhealthy situation even worse. Imagine the little clot-encrusted pieces cracking off and lodging downstream in smaller arteries, which can easily be blocked.

So where does this long, complicated story about your atoms and molecules end? As we said earlier, NO molecules help prevent heart attacks and strokes by relaxing your blood vessels and keeping them soft, elastic, and open. NO reduces inflammation, not only in the blood vessels, but anywhere in the body where the inflammation may be present. That's basically how NO reduces the risk of chronic degenerative diseases (see pg. 78).

Let's consider another example of the scientific wonders of NO. Dr. Carl Nathan, of Cornell University, recently uncovered another amazing dimension of the NO Paradigm. His research shows that when inflammation is *not* present in the human body, it's not because there are no injuries, infections, or threats. Dr. Nathan discovered that if your body is not inflamed, it's not just because it's your body's normal passive state. This means maintaining health requires steady, positive actions to suppress the body's continuous reactions to threats that are always present. Thus, in the NO Paradigm, wellness is more than just the absence of disease. *It depends on steady, positive action.* This is why we prescribe **The Wellness Solution**.

Miraculously, even the most dimly lit pilot light in your body can still be ignited by producing more NO. So, in summary, the NO Paradigm Shift is a complete U-turn in the way you think about health: It's all about taking steps to support NO in your body through a healthy daily routine . . . **The Wellness Solution**.

We are honored that you have taken the time to read this far. Now we would like you to take full advantage of the latest research and the therapeutic benefits of our patient-physician partnership. In the final pages that follow, we invite you to join us and create a new symphony for your atoms so your physical, psychological, and spiritual resources can get in perfect harmony. We call this . . . **molecular wellness.**

It's as if Walt Whitman had NO in mind when he wrote the following stanzas in *Leaves of Grass.*

> *You will hardly know who I am, or what I mean;*
> *But I shall be good health to you nevertheless,*
> *and filter and fiber your blood.*
> *Failing to find me at first, keep encouraged;*
> *Missing me one place, search another;*
> *I stop somewhere, waiting for you.*

Molecular Wellness

Dr. Ferid Murad is awarded the Albert Lasker Award for Basic Medical Research "for having advanced the fundamental understanding of biochemical mechanisms in cells."

—Inscription Accompanying the
Highest Medical Award in the United States

The wise physician today recognizes that the physiological, psychological, and spiritual resources of the patient are an important part of the total strategy of treatment, along with the best that modern medical science has to offer. Dr. Edward Taub's clinical research provides an up-to-date guide to putting the patient's own resources to work, and in so doing, he makes full use of the latest research in the concept of the patient-physician partnership."

—Norman Cousins, Author, *Anatomy of an Illness*

Taub-Murad-Oliphant Medical Research Associates, our professional partnership, is engaged in the practice of Integrative Medicine, the fastest-growing health field in America. Integrative Medicine means joining responsible self-care and holistic practices with the very best resources and practices that modern medicine has to offer.

We write from the perspective of two wellness medical doctors and a uniquely well-informed patient, who are committed to providing world-class wellness care for everyone. As a patient, you have the right to expect that our recommendations are scientific and will do no harm. In return, we promise that what has been written in this book will not betray your trust.

We look at this book as a health guide for our practice. Our practice is strictly an advisory medical practice that shares knowledge with you. But medical knowledge is powerful only when patients know how to act upon it. And all our sound advice is worth nothing unless you are inspired to put it into use. Therefore, to motivate you, we've combined our work and vision to create a practice unlike any other, anywhere. It's based on attaining **molecular wellness.**

Our advice is not intended as a substitute for having a personal physician who has examined you and is familiar with your history. Integrative Medicine, by definition, is a complement to proper medical diagnosis and care. We hope to make you a very well-informed patient!

Health care is not what it used to be. Today, doctors spend less and less time with patients, and most health insurance companies are more concerned with profits than with your well-being. On the other hand, many patients demand expensive new drugs, now advertised on TV, that provide no better relief and cause far more side effects. Consider the mind-boggling fact that roughly 80 percent of all new drugs introduced in the last 20 years offer no significant advantage over drugs they have replaced, even though they are astronomically more expensive. Many Americans take so many prescription drugs that if it weren't so alarming, it would just be ridiculous. The present health care system is financially out of control, and too many patients participate in it at their grave risk. Excellence and integrity are no longer its guiding principles. Profit is paramount. Why else would the executives of health care organizations be making astronomical incomes?

Your health, we wholeheartedly believe, is more determined by what you are willing to do for yourself, rather than what the present health care system is able to do for you. Attaining molecular wellness is the key, and it is the ideal state of health we are striving for with all our patients. If you agree, then we extend our hand to you in a therapeutic partnership you can count on.

As we have said many times, health is your most precious asset, and as your wellness doctors, we can help you with beneficial information that might otherwise be wasted while physicians and the medical establishment catch up with the cutting-edge scientific knowledge about NO. But your compliance with *The Wellness Solution* is crucial. It's a proven way to take better, more scientifically responsible care of yourself. Let's repeat it. . . . Compliance is crucial, not optional.

Wellness Theology

You can have tens of millions of dollars, but what does it mean if you're ill as a result of low NO levels in your body? This is why we repeatedly remind you that health is your most precious asset, worth more than anything you could ever buy. Isn't that enough to motivate you to invest a serious effort in complying with *The Wellness Solution*?

There are two major reasons why your health and wellness depend so much on your resolve to fully comply with the TLC (therapeutic lifestyle changes) that form the basis of *The Wellness Solution*.

First of all, each component of *The Wellness Solution* is part of a live symphony in which your own physical, psychological, and spiritual energies are brought into perfect harmony with one another.

That's the ultimate definition of molecular wellness.

Secondly, left to its own devices, your mind will probably resist behaving healthfully. It will find every excuse available not to exercise, and probably even invent a few new ones. Your mind also won't be anxious to deny the urgent calls of your appetite and taste buds. The key is to get your body producing more NO immediately! You'll feel much better because of higher NO levels, and in return the increased NO will drive your healthy behavior to keep up the good feeling. This NO biofeedback loop offers some really wonderful consequences. Things can automatically fall into place, and new habits can take off on their own, because NO molecules function as neurotransmitters, conveying wellness messages back and forth between the body and brain.

The NO Paradigm is a joyful, uplifting paradigm of wellness, not illness. Time and time again, we've observed that patients with a positive outlook and a sense of humor do better than their more negative-minded counterparts.

Newly published research has shown how laughter can increase production of NO to help relax the blood vessels and lower blood pressure. No wonder it's been reported that people who laugh frequently have fewer heart attacks than people less inclined to see humor in everyday events! Overall, it appears that the happier you are, the more NO you'll produce . . . and the more NO you produce, the happier you feel. How happy does that make you?

Faith, hope, and prayer are also essential cornerstones for building health and overall well-being. Harvard Medical School's Dr. Herbert Benson teaches medical students and physicians that faith, hope, and prayer increase the body's production of NO. From a spiritual standpoint, India's Sathya Sai Baba teaches that if you take one genuine step toward God, then God takes one thousand steps toward you. Or, if you cry one genuine tear, God wipes away ten thousand. This powerful combination of scientific and spiritual considerations is something we think is best referred to as "Wellness Theology."

Dr. Jonas Salk's Living Legacy

Americans can only hope that Dr. Edward Taub will expand his research and develop a wellness vaccination to inoculate our minds and bodies against stress. I look forward to a vaccination without needles and with all its side effects being positive!

—Jonas Salk, M.D., Polio Vaccine Pioneer

Dr. Ferid Murad knew nitroglycerine caused relaxation of smooth muscle cells. The enzyme, guanylyl cyclase, was activated and increased cyclic GMP, causing relaxation of the muscle. Did nitroglycerin act via release of Nitric Oxide? Dr. Murad bubbled Nitric Oxide gas through tissue containing the enzyme. Cyclic GMP increased! A new mode of drug action had been discovered!

—Inscription Accompanying the
Nobel Prize in Medicine

The story of the NO Paradigm is one of the greatest health stories since Dr. Jonas Salk's polio vaccination. We believe *The Wellness Solution* is Dr. Salk's living legacy, because it has the potential to do as much good as his famous vaccine.

Fifty years ago, experts proclaimed that Dr. Salk's polio vaccination couldn't possibly be effective. Why not? Because the prevailing wisdom indicated that dead-virus vaccines could not work. Yet Dr. Salk's vaccine, made from dead viruses, prevailed. Needless to say, it also triggered a major health paradigm discovery!

Over 25 years ago, in 1980, after learning about Dr. Edward Taub's pioneering work in wellness and Integrative Medicine, Dr. Salk urged him to develop a wellness vaccine.

Subsequently, in a presentation to the Institute of Medicine in Washington, D.C., Dr. Taub reported the results of his wellness program, based on over 2,000 patients in his group medical practice. The doctors in the program significantly reduced illness and medical costs by dispensing health information, along with a new health philosophy. Patients were informed, and then reminded at each office visit, that their health was mostly determined by their own personal responsibility, self-value, and reverence for life. They were taught about the importance of managing stress, including being a good person. They also learned about healthy nutrition, weight management, vitamins and minerals, and the wisdom of drinking adequate amounts of water and exercising regularly.

The medical school deans in the audience that day in Washington, D.C., applauded Dr. Taub's vision of Integrative Medicine, but lamented the fact that when they presented this type of information to medical students, the budding doctors usually tuned out and dozed off. One dean actually called it "The Big Sleep." Since the 1980s, Integrative Medicine has grown immensely and is now part of the standard curriculum in many medical schools across the country. Even so, it is safe to say that the vast majority of medical students and practicing physicians have failed to take Integrative Medicine very seriously. These trained skeptics continue to be hesitant because scientific explanations for Integrative Medicine's effectiveness have been a lot "softer" than doctors might traditionally prefer.

But there is nothing soft about the recent research findings we've shared with you. . . . These reports should send a giant wake-up call to medical students and practicing physicians alike. "The Big Sleep" is over! No doctor can afford to ignore what the president of the American Heart Association foresaw in 1998 when commenting on Dr. Murad's Nobel Prize. He said, "The discovery of NO and its function is one of the most important in the history of cardiovascular medicine." Now we know there is even much more to NO. So, doctors, if you're snoozing during this lesson, you're missing some of the most significant information of your education!

We have uncovered the true scientific basis for Integrative Medicine . . . **molecular wellness.** Essentially, we've identified a new mode of drug action in which therapeutic lifestyle changes stimulate the body's own internal healing pharmacy. For the first time, a wide body of scientific information supports TLC! Thus, it seems very appropriate to commemorate the 50th anniversary of Dr. Salk's contribution to humanity with a new, revolutionary wellness vaccination . . . *The Wellness Solution*. Dr. Salk would be happy to know his vision of a wellness inoculation has in fact happened!

The Taub-Murad-Oliphant Syndrome

New doors of understanding and opportunities for healing and prevention are opened up when you recognize that heart attacks and strokes are not just plumbing problems caused by a buildup of fat in the vessels that lead to the heart and brain. The underlying problem is inflammation, which also poisons the rest of the body, leading to the wide array of chronic degenerative diseases summarized in the chart on page 78.

We have emphasized that inflammation has a purpose as a natural healing response. It's the body's attempt to protect and eventually heal itself. However, in our current times, injury, infection, and threats are constant consequences of insufficient levels of NO. As a result, hundreds of millions of bodies, mainly in the United States and other "highly developed" nations, are rusting away with oxidative stress, being infiltrated with fat, and suffering with GH and Simmering Stress Syndrome. This leads to ongoing inflammation and chronic degenerative diseases as a result of too little NO. We believe the situation can be avoided. How? You can now answer that question yourself, from what you have read so far in this book.

We call this complex disease condition the Taub-Murad-Oliphant Syndrome (TMO Syndrome, or Rampant Entropy). It is widespread throughout the entire developed world, especially in the United States. **In a nutshell, the TMO Syndrome is an abnormal prevalent state in**

the body in which the force of entropy (degeneration) is triumphing over the force of homeostasis (healing). Put simply, in this state, the body is deteriorating prematurely. This form of rampant entropy interferes with and dramatically speeds up the normal human life cycle. It appears destined to be the scourge of the 21st century.

Do you have the TMO Syndrome? If you are significantly overweight, chronically stressed out, not taking a comprehensive vitamin and mineral supplement, and experiencing a form of chronic degenerative disease, then you almost certainly have it. If you also have a high C-reactive protein level, that pretty much confirms the diagnosis. Are there beginning and intermediate stages? Of course there are. This is not a gloom-and-doom report. We wrote this book to help you reduce your risk of these degenerative diseases.

The TMO Syndrome is a complex disorder and an emerging clinical challenge, and we look forward to the help many medical experts can provide for specific diagnostic guidelines in the future. In the meantime, since there are no well-accepted, established criteria for the diagnosis of the TMO Syndrome, you'll pretty much have to be your own diagnostician and use your common sense. We suggest you have a complete physical examination and discuss the TMO Syndrome with your personal physician.

Please believe that we are not trying to scare you, but it's important for you to realize that unless effective steps are taken to stop its progress, the TMO Syndrome inevitably leads to deterioration. The good news is that it can be slowed down or reversed in most cases! The key to prevention and treatment of the TMO Syndrome is producing more NO. That's where *The Wellness Solution* comes in, big time!

The Wellness Solution is the key to molecular wellness, which is the other side of the molecular medicine coin that usually concentrates on illness, not wellness. More than just the absence of disease, wellness is homeostasis and entropy in balance at various stages of the human life cycle—our youth, our reproductive years, and our nurturing and aging years. To achieve molecular wellness is to reach the point of balance in which physical, psychological, and spiritual energies are so finely attuned to one another that distinctions between them fade away. It's a process of natural healing, not necessarily curing. It's when you are feeling at your peak, or maybe experiencing a "eureka" moment of great insight or a true epiphany. It's when, even in the process of dying, we can experience freedom from fear, comforted by knowing we are part of something much greater than ourselves.

The prevention and cure of the TMO Syndrome is triggered by an increased production of NO molecules—your own internal healing pharmacy. Then, in a natural biofeedback loop, wellness itself triggers even more production of NO molecules. Can you see how this is truly homeostasis at its wondrous best?

Imagine messages carried by "puffs" of NO gas providing the Spark of Life throughout your body to stave off or treat chronic degenerative diseases. Imagine NO molecules bolstering your immune system; protecting your heart, blood vessel, and brain health; combating stress hormones; enhancing memory; and even helping a flagging libido. *The Wellness Solution*, which is the treatment for the TMO Syndrome, is like Viagra for the entire body.

Most Americans currently live in a paradigm based on illness, not wellness. Drugs, surgery, and radiation are hallmarks of the old paradigm. NO is the focal point of the new health care paradigm, so our treatment plan focuses on helping your body to produce more NO. It will never do you harm, and it is a wonderful adjunct to the ongoing care of your personal physician.

Surgeon, Heal Thyself

"It's too difficult," were the words heard from another physician during the last week of writing this book. We ran into a trauma surgeon at the hospital. More precisely, he ran into us as he dashed around a corner on the way to the operating room. It was alarming to see how hassled and stressed he was. We caught up with one another, during a slower moment, later that day in the doctors' dining room.

The surgeon asked what we were up to. We shared our work on this book and suggested that *The Wellness Solution* would be perfect for him. He shared our enthusiasm, but when it came to following *The Wellness Solution* himself, he replied, "It's too difficult." That remark stayed in our minds because we realize that health is our most precious asset.

Between finishing off a 16-ounce soft drink and ordering a mocha malt coffee with whipped cream from the coffee kiosk, the surgeon in the dining room said to us, "I know, I know, I know. . . . I should be taking better care of myself. To tell you the truth, I've been getting severe chest pains since my wife died six months ago. That's probably a sign of heart damage, so I've put off seeing a doctor, because I'm dreading what I might learn. My wife died recently, and I really loved her. We were childhood sweethearts. So I guess I just don't want to deal with more bad news."

As the surgeon pointed to the open white coat he couldn't button over his abdomen, he continued, "Look, I know what you want to tell me, but I don't have time for exercise and it's not easy to eat right when I'm always on the run. But my God, my weight gain has been staggering! I'm 50 years old, and I'm already 50 pounds heavier than when I graduated medical school 25 years ago!"

Sounding almost combative, the surgeon continued, "Look, I wouldn't even know where to get started on taking vitamins. I was taught that if I take vitamins, they just wind up in the urine because we get enough from what we eat—except, I suppose, if you eat a lot of junk food like I do."

"Oh, and as far as stress is concerned," he exclaimed, "forget about it! Have you seen how many auto-accident victims wind up in this hospital every day, and the shape that they're in? I mean, where am I going to get time for meditation or prayer—in the bathroom between operations?"

Then, suddenly dejected, the surgeon said, "I know, I know, I've got to make time and I've got to take better care of myself. But it's too difficult."

We haven't spoken with the surgeon since then. He's been too busy. But he's a real poster child, if you will, for TMO Syndrome. His sad, misguided statement sticks with you: *"It's too difficult."*

When the doctor does make up his mind to slow down for a moment, we'd like to tell him about a few of the amazing studies that have recently been published, because scientists all over the world are contributing to a virtual avalanche of research relating to NO that should inspire even the most disheartened and disillusioned individual to understand. . . . It's time to get on board with *The Wellness Solution*!

The Broken Heart Syndrome

In 2005, researchers discovered that profound emotional shock, such as the loss of a loved one, can literally break your heart. Such stressful news has long been thought to cause heart attacks. However, researchers at the Johns Hopkins University School of Medicine have discovered that this type of profound emotional stress can also result in severe—but reversible—heart muscle weakness that *mimics* a classic heart attack.

This is the broken heart syndrome. This new syndrome is a significant reason for the chest pains and heart attacks that doctors see every day in emergency rooms, but may not be diagnosing correctly.

Patients who have lost a loved one can be misdiagnosed with a heart attack when instead they are suffering from a prolonged surge of stress hormones that temporarily stun their heart muscles. Earlier in the book, we suggested that being "ill" could sometimes be synonymous with "I lack love."

Chest pains and heartache following the lost of a loved one is a medical condition known as stress cardiomyopathy. Researchers at Johns Hopkins found that the levels of stress hormones in patients with the broken heart syndrome were wildly elevated. This is a dramatic example of the Simmering Stress Syndrome boiling over, leading to symptoms similar to a severe heart attack.

We wonder whether the surgeon's chest pains since his wife's death are due to the broken heart syndrome. In any case, we'd like to tell the surgeon he'd better get on the ball by increasing his NO, starting with our Emergency Stress Treatment, so he can stay out of the emergency room as a patient. This treatment, designed for ER doctors in the stressful days after 9/11, is an effective prescription for quieting minds. He should know that preventing or treating the TMO Syndrome is not too difficult.

Supplements Are Important

Our surgeon friend, like almost all medical doctors, was taught in medical school that patients who are taking nutritional supplements are merely enriching their urine. Such statements ignore the Generalized Hypovitaminosis Syndrome we have identified and explained earlier. He is also missing the fact that research now shows that even if patients eat very well, it is highly unlikely they will get the vitamins and minerals that science shows can help reduce the risk of major diseases when used along with *The Wellness Solution*. That's why a landmark review in the *Journal of the American Medical Association* in 2002 concludes that it is prudent for all adults to take a vitamin and mineral supplement every day! Of course, there are no magic pills for the surgeon or for his patients. That's why we recommend taking a scientifically balanced vitamin and mineral system (see page 63), but only as part of an overall strategy to eat healthfully, manage weight, drink appropriate amounts of water, exercise regularly, not smoke, and manage stress, which includes being a good person. This is *The Wellness Solution*.

The good news is that following *The Wellness Solution*, in conjunction with proper medical treatment, can help reverse endothelial dysfunction and result in increased levels of NO. We particularly want our surgeon friend to know that supplementation with the proper amounts of vitamins and minerals, especially antioxidants, can improve NO production in his body.

Save Your Life from a Fat Attack . . . . More Good Information

One of the more troubling things about the surgeon's health state was his obesity. In 2005, a first-of-its-kind analysis published in the *New England Journal of Medicine* determined that illnesses caused by obesity shorten the average American's lifespan more than the impact of car accidents, homicides, and suicides combined. If the trend is not reversed, obesity will take a greater toll on the average American's lifespan than even cancer! "It's sort of like a massive tsunami heading toward the shoreline," said Dr. David S. Ludwig, an obesity expert at Harvard Medical School and Children's Hospital in Boston.

The public health care crisis over obesity is part of the larger crisis of the TMO Syndrome. In an editorial that accompanied the above article in the *New England Journal of Medicine,* Dr. Samuel Preston points out that, while 67 percent of American adults are now overweight, the recent increases in the levels of obesity in America are caused by *relatively few* excess calories in the typical daily diet. How many? Hold on to your hat!

The consumption of an average of just 30 excess calories a day is responsible for the typical weight gain of adults between 20 and 40 years old. This can certainly account for the 50 pounds the surgeon gained over the last 25 years, since graduating medical school. This means the doctor could put the breaks on getting even fatter by cutting down on some of his 16-ounce regular cola soft drinks (200 calories) or whipped cream and coffee concoctions (500 to 800 calories). There is hope for all of us, if we cut down on calories, just here and there. That said, a combination of calorie reduction, increased exercise, and boosting NO makes it all happen. Just remember, simple common sense offers all of us great hope. Our motto is, *Everything in moderation . . . including moderation!*

The overall picture should be clear enough for even the surgeon to see. Simmering stress and excess fat lead to rust and inflammation, which eventually lead to chronic degenerative diseases. The doctor has a classic case of the TMO Syndrome. On the other hand, even this extremely stressed-out surgeon can help save his life by following ***The Wellness Solution***.

Everything in Moderation . . . Including Moderation. It's Not Too Difficult!

To sum it up, our mission and prescription is to help you avoid illness. If you are currently ill, our genuine desire is to help you on your journey to wellness, safely and quickly. Our gift to you is ***The Wellness Solution***, which will boost NO and promote molecular wellness. All that we ask for in return is your compliance and trust. Follow ***The Wellness Solution***, have trust in God, trust in yourself, and trust in the best scientific information we have presented in the book.

The foundation that awards the Nobel Prize in Medicine wisely recognized the discovery of NO as a signaling molecule in the body. We are privileged to have identified NO as the Spark of Life. Our final prescription comes right from our heart. . . . Follow *The Wellness Solution*, be happy, laugh, and increase your NO and life expectancy.

A PERSONAL NOTE FROM . . .

David Oliphant

Being part of such a prestigious team as publisher and co-author of *The Wellness Solution* has been a true labor of love. Let me explain why.

As you read in the foreword, one of my most satisfying personal achievements in life has been my involvement with the Leukemia & Lymphoma Society of America for over 30 years. Helping people and giving of yourself, I feel, is one of the most important contributions any human being can make to the world, especially if you are in a position to do so. This book represents, to me, that same achievement. I hope that millions of people will read *The Wellness Solution* because there is so much invaluable information that will help people attain optimal health and become well-informed patients.

Dr. Taub and Dr. Murad call me the "well-informed patient." That's probably a subject for another book, but in the meantime, yes, I've made myself a very well-informed patient, because in these times, when doctors are so busy and have less and less time to give us, it's important that we do everything possible to stay well in the first place. That is the goal of wellness and preventive medicine.

Many times throughout the book you have read the disclaimer and suggestion to always check with your doctor before taking the advice or recommendations that have been offered. I'm sure you must have said to yourself, "Wow, they surely are protecting themselves!" Well, you're right, but there's another side of the coin. We truly believe that *The Wellness Solution* is designed for you to work with your personal physician. It would be irresponsible of Dr. Taub or Dr. Murad to give you blanket advice without meeting you personally, examining you, and getting your medical and family history.

Before closing, I want to mention that my blessings in life have been numerous. My most precious blessing was when I married Deborah Ann Kalman over 18 years ago. Our relationship is truly my greatest achievement in love and in life.

Finally, I would like to share with you two of Dr. Taub's famous sayings, which were my first lesson in becoming a well-informed patient:

"Everything in moderation . . . including moderation!"
and
"Your health is your most precious asset!"

Remember, this book is an incredible guide to a healthier you!

Wishing you good health,

David Oliphant

Ferid Murad, M.D., Ph.D.

It has been such a pleasure to work with Dr. Edward Taub and David Oliphant on this book. Since the project began with some discussions about one and a half years ago, I have learned so much more about the elements of *The Wellness Solution*—a way for patients to take charge of their preventive medicine and health care. Dr. Taub opened my eyes to numerous ways to enhance Nitric Oxide production and function. Who would have thought in 1977, when we first discovered the first biological effects of a toxic pollutant gas—Nitric Oxide—to relax smooth muscle, that the field would virtually explode into numerous areas of biology and medicine over the past two and a half decades? Numerous drugs have been developed from our research and that of others in this field, and many more are to be discovered for a multitude of disorders. To learn that even laughter increases Nitric Oxide formation and lowers blood pressure amazes me but shouldn't surprise me. After all, there have been about 100,000 publications in the field of NO research since our first publications in 1977. This area of biology seems to be producing more amazing announcements all the time.

The writing of this book has improved the lifestyle and behavior of a workaholic scientist: me. I have even found myself increasing my use of vitamins and antioxidants after seeing some of the convincing publications we found while preparing this book.

As a physician and a scientist, there is nothing more gratifying than to see your work benefit millions of people. Hopefully, millions more can benefit by following the recommendations in this book.

While Dr. Taub and I approached *The Wellness Solution* and the Generalized Hypovitaminosis Syndrome from different directions—he from his clinical practice and interest in Integrative Medicine, and I from the biochemistry and pharmacology of Nitric Oxide—we rapidly came to similar conclusions and developed a common language. In science we would call that a very significant accomplishment, when the same conclusions are reached while coming at a problem from different directions.

Should there be another edition to this book in a year or two, and I suspect there will be, I am sure there will be another 5,000 to 10,000 scientific publications on Nitric Oxide to digest for our readers. I look forward to a continued relationship with Dr. Edward Taub and David Oliphant and another book assignment.

Here's to keeping your Nitric Oxide levels elevated and remaining healthy. And remember to laugh when you can. . . . It's healthy!

Ferid Murad, M.D., Ph.D.

Edward A. Taub, M.D.

Dr. Murad has an unparalleled scientific mind, and together we have combined intuition with theoretical and empirical judgment to identify NO as the Spark of Life and prescribe *The Wellness Solution*.

David Oliphant recognized the value of *The Wellness Solution* when it was in its infancy, and he nurtured it to maturity. I urge you to re-read his Foreword to appreciate why the wisdom that you've glimpsed in this book cannot be easily forgotten.

When I founded The Wellness Medical Institute, my licensed medical practice, to respond to a challenge by Dr. Jonas Salk, I could not have known that I would wait another 25 years for Dr. Ferid Murad's and Dave Oliphant's help to reach my goal.

I'll explain by first sharing an incredible coincidence. While getting ready to write this personal note, I happened to glance at a newspaper headline announcing that it was the 50th anniversary of a time when Americans overcame their greatest fear, when the news of Dr. Salk's polio vaccination was officially released in two simple sentences: "The vaccine works. It is safe, effective, and potent."

Let's go back in time. . . . In another coincidence, that announcement, which electrified America, was made on the 10th anniversary of President Franklin D. Roosevelt's death. The president, already crippled by polio, had greatly comforted Americans during the horror of World War II by proclaiming, "The only thing we have to fear is fear itself." Ironically, after the end of the war, polio became the worst nightmare imaginable. By then, Americans were afraid of an imminent nuclear attack from Russia, and every child had to do "duck-and-seek-cover" drills under their desks at school. But Americans were even more afraid of polio. Horrifying epidemics arrived each summer, killing thousands of children and paralyzing tens of thousands more. Movie theaters and swimming pools were closed. Newspapers published daily counts of new victims, along with pictures of pitiful children struggling with crutches. There were also fearful pictures of rows of patients in iron lung machines in vast hospital wards.

Fortunately, President Roosevelt organized the National Foundation for Infantile Paralysis, now known as the March of Dimes, to conquer polio, and that led to Dr. Salk's great contribution to humanity. At a ceremony in the White House, President Eisenhower said to Dr. Salk, "I have no words to thank you. I am very, very happy."

"Who owns the patent on this vaccine?" asked Edward R. Murrow, the famous news reporter. Doctor Salk responded, "Well, the people, I would say. There is no patent. Could you patent the sun?"

Dr. Salk had stuck with his belief in a dead-virus vaccine, even though the notion was widely ridiculed by most other scientists of the time. They believed that only a live-virus vaccine could possibly work. Talk about a paradigm shift! Dr. Salk's enduring message to all scientists was to think differently if we intend to conquer the major scourges of humanity.

Twenty-five years later, after reviewing my clinical research with over 2,000 patients, Dr. Salk personally challenged me to think differently. Specifically, he challenged me to develop a wellness vaccination to benefit humanity. Since my major skill has always been with patient care rather than with laboratory research, I founded The Wellness Medical Institute, to practice Integrative Medicine and create a wellness inoculation. As I said before, I could not have known that I would wait another 25 years for Dr. Ferid Murad's and Dave Oliphant's help to realize my goal.

Both David Oliphant and his wife, Deborah Kalman Oliphant, have been beside me for over a decade, helping me tell the world about wellness. It's impossible not to be moved by their hard work, decency, and sincerity. Now they have helped to identify as well as to tell the story of *The Wellness Solution*.

Dr. Ferid Murad is a spectacularly brilliant, accomplished, and caring physician and pharmacologist. Remember, before winning the Nobel

Prize, he won the Albert Lasker Award for Basic Medical Research, the highest achievement in American medicine, *"for having advanced the fundamental understanding of biochemical mechanisms in cells."*

I'm honored that Dr. Murad agrees with the premises and conclusions I've reached in my clinical experience with patients. Indeed, he has added substantially to my work and brought closure to Dr. Salk's challenge to develop a wellness vaccination. It's *The Wellness Solution*.

In his personal note, Dr. Murad suggests that updated editions of this book may occur over the years. Indeed, I envision a series of books on Integrative Medicine, perhaps *Wellness Pediatrics, Wellness Psychiatry, Wellness Obstetrics and Gynecology,* and *Wellness Geriatrics.* We'll see.

In the meantime, by following the easy-to-use guidelines of *The Wellness Solution*, you can be assured of the happiest, healthiest life possible. When I first took the Hippocratic oath, I pledged to practice medicine with conscience and dignity, holding my patients' trust as sacred. I also promised to do all within my power to help my patients attain physical, mental, and spiritual health. NO adds a new dimension and helps me fulfill my pledge, because NO is not only the molecular basis of wellness and the Spark of Life, it's also equivalent to God's presence in each of our cells. Helping you discover something so exceptional has required a great deal of research and storytelling on our parts. It has also required a great deal of dedication to the truth on your part. By following *The Wellness Solution* . . . your journey to a healthier life has surely begun.

Edward A. Taub, M.D.

THE WELLNESS SOLUTION
RESOURCES FOR PHYSICIANS

The purpose of this resource section is to put the emerging area of Nitric Oxide investigation for the prevention and treatment of chronic degenerative diseases into focus, to provide physicians with a new armamentarium for patient care. Interpreting the logic and methodology of our scientific inquiry will hopefully assist physicians to construct a more meaningful balance between the art and science of medicine.

SELECTED BIBLIOGRAPHY

Benson, Herbert, M.D. *The Breakout Principle*. Scribner, 2003.

Bohm, David, Ph.D. *Wholeness and Implicate Order*. Routledge and Kegan Paul, 1980.

Buber, Martin, Ph.D. *I and Thou*. Scribner, 1958.

Chopra, Deepak, M.D. *Ageless Body, Timeless Mind*. Harmony, 1993.

Cooke, John P., M.D., Ph.D. *The Cardiovascular Cure*. Broadway Books, 2002.

Cousins, Norman. *Anatomy of an Illness*. Norton, 1979.

Damasio, Antonio R., M.D. *Descartes' Error*. Grosset/Putman, 1994.

Diamond, Harvey, and Marilyn Diamond. *Fit for Life*. Warner, 1985.

Dossey, Larry, M.D. *Healing Words*. HarperCollins, 1993.

Emerson, Ralph Waldo. *Self Reliance* (1841). Kessinger Publishing, 2005.

Frankl, Victor E., M.D. *Man's Search for Meaning*. Washington Square Press, 1959.

Goleman, Daniel P., Ph.D. *Emotional Intelligence*. Bantam Books, 2005.

Groopman, Jerome, M.D. *The Anatomy of Hope: How People Prevail in the Face of Illness*. Random House, 2003.

Hesse, Herman. *Siddhartha*. Bantam, 1951.

James, William, M.D. *Principles of Psychology: Volume One*. Dover Publications, 1950.

Joy, Brugh, M.D. *Joy's Way*. Putnam Books, 1979.

Murad, Ferid, M.D., Ph.D. *Nitric Oxide: Biochemistry, Molecular Biology, and Therapeutic Implications*. (Advances in Pharmacology, Vol.34). Academic Press, 1995.

————. *Discovery of Some of the Biological Effects of Nitric Oxide and Its Role in Cell Signaling*. Le Prix Nobel, 1998.

Ornish, Dean, M.D. *Dr. Dean Ornish's Program for Reversing Heart Disease*. Random House, 1990.

Pelletier, Kenneth, Ph.D. *Mind as Healer, Mind as Slayer*. Delacorte Press, 1977.

Sandweiss, Samuel H., M.D. *Sai Baba: The Holy Man and the Psychiatrist*. Birthday Press, 1995.

Schuller, Robert H., Ph.D. *Self-Esteem: The New Reformation.* Word Books, 1982.

Schweitzer, Albert, M.D. *Out of My Life and Thought: An Autobiography.* The Johns Hopkins University Press, 1998.

Slobody, Lawrence B., M.D., and David Oliphant. *A 12-Step Anti-Aging Plan for a Longer, Healthier & Happier Life.* Bergin & Garvey, 1996.

Taub, Edward A., M.D. *Balance Your Body, Balance Your Life.* Pocket Books, 1999.

————. *The Seven Steps to Self Healing.* DK Publishing, 1996.

Valliant, George E., Ph.D. *The Wisdom of the Ego.* Harvard, 1993.

Veith, Ilza, trans. *The Yellow Emperor's Classic of Internal Medicine.* University of California Press, 1949.

Williamson, Marianne. *A Return to Love.* HarperCollins, 1992.

Wilson, Edward O., Ph.D. *Consilience: The Unity of Knowledge.* Alfred A. Knopf, 1998.

SELECTED REFERENCES

Ad Hoc Committee to Defend Health Care. "For our patients, not for profits: A call to action." *Journal of the American Medical Association* 278 (1997): 1733–1740.

Leaf, Alexander, M.D., and T. J. Ryan, M.D. "Prevention of coronary artery disease: A medical imperative." *New England Journal of Medicine* 323 (1990): 1416–1419.

Moncada, Salvador. "Nitric oxide: Discovery and impact on clinical medicine." *Journal of the Royal Society of Medicine* 92 (1999): 164–169.

Moncada, Salvador, and Annie Higgs, a review article. "Mechanisms of disease: The L-arginine–nitric oxide pathway." *New England Journal of Medicine* 329 (1993): 2002–2012.

Murad, Ferid, M.D., Ph.D. "The Discovery of Some of the Biological Effects of Nitric Oxide and Its Role in Cell Signaling" (The Nobel Lecture, 1998).

———. "The excitement and rewards of research with our discovery of some of the biological effects of nitric oxide." *Circulation Research* 92 (2003): 339–341.

———. "Nitric oxide signaling: Would you believe that a simple free radical could be a second messenger, autocoid, paracrine substance, neurotransmitter, and hormone?" *Recent Progress in Hormone Research* 53 (1998): 43–60.

Robert Wood Johnson Foundation. *Chronic Care in America: A 21st Century Challenge.* Princeton, 1996.

Taub, Edward A., M.D. "Wellness paradigm shift." *Mind/Body Medicine: A Journal of Clinical Behavioral Medicine,* Vol. 1, No.2 (1995): 82–84.

Wells, William, Ph.D. "From explosives to the gas that heals: Nitric oxide in biology and medicine." *Beyond Discovery: The Path from Research to Human Benefit.* National Academy of Sciences, 2001.

NITRIC OXIDE (NO) AND ENDOTHELIAL HEALTH

Altman, L. "Three Americans Share Nobel Prize in Medicine," *New York Times,* October 13, 1998.

Canto, J. G., and A. A. Iskandrian, editorial. "Major risk factors for cardiovascular disease debunking the 'Only 50%' Myth." *Journal of the American Medical Association* 290 (2003): 947–949.

Charikida, M. et al. "The role of nitric oxide in early atherosclerosis." *European Journal of Clinical Pharmacology.* Suppl. no. 13 (2005): 69–77.

Greenland, P. et al. "Major risk factors as antecedents of fatal and nonfatal coronary heart disease events." *Journal of the American Medical Association* 290 (2003): 891–897.

Hackam, D. G., and S. S. Anand. "Emerging risk factors for atherosclerotic vascular disease: A critical review of the evidence." *Journal of the American Medical Association* 290 (2003): 932–940.

Heatherton and Renn. "Stress and the disinhibition of behavior." *Mind/Body Medicine: A Journal of Clinical Behavioral Medicine,* Vol. 1, No.2 (1997): 72–81.

Khot, U. N. et al. "Prevalence of conventional risk factors in patients with coronary heart disease." *Journal of the American Medical Association* 290 (2003): 898–904.

Murad, Ferid, M.D., Ph.D. "Cyclic GMP synthesis, metabolism and function." *Advances in Pharmacology* 26 (1994): 1–335.

———. "Cyclic guanosine monophosphate as a mediator of vasodilation." *Journal of Clinical Investigation* 78 (1986): 1–5.

———. "Drugs used in the treatment of angina: Organic nitrites, calcium channel blockers and adrenergic antagonists." *The Pharmacological Basis of Therapeutics* VIII Edition (1990): 764–783.

———. *Nitric Oxide: Biochemistry, Molecular Biology, and Therapeutic Implications.* (Advances in Pharmacology, Vol.34). Academic Press, 1995.

———. "Nitric oxide signaling: Would you believe that a simple free radical could be a second messenger, autocoid, paracrine substance, neurotransmitter, and hormone?" *Recent Progress in Hormone Research* 53 (1998): 43–60.

———. "Signal transduction using nitric oxide and cyclic guanosine monophosphate." *Journal of the American Medical Association* 276 (1996): 1189–1192.

Taub, Edward A., M.D. *Seven Steps to Self Healing.* DK Publishing, 1998.

———. *The Wellness Rx.* Prentice Hall, 1994.

Tousoulis, D. et al. "Endothelial function and inflammation in coronary artery disease." *Heart* 92 (2006): 441–444.

Widlansky, M. E. et al. The clinical implications of endothelial dysfunction. *Journal of the American College of Cardiology* 42 (2003): 1149–1160.

GENERALIZED HYPOVITAMINOSIS

Age-Related Eye Disease Research Group. "A randomized, placebo-controlled, clinical trial of high-dose supplementation with vitamins C and E, beta carotene, and zinc for age-related macular degeneration and vision loss." *Archives of Ophthalmology* 119 (2001): 1417–1436.

Beckman, K. B., and B. N. Ames. "Free radical theory of aging matures." *Physiological Reviews* 78 (1998): 547–581.

Carr, A., and B. Frei. "The role of natural antioxidants in preserving the biological activity of endothelium-derived nitric oxide." *Free Radic Biol Med* 28 (2000): 1806–1814.

Chandra, R. K. "Graying of the immune system: Can nutrient supplements improve immunity in the elderly?" *Journal of the American Medical Association* 227 (1997): 1398–1399.

Fawzi, W., and M. J. Stampfer, editorial. "A role for multivitamins in infection?" *Annals of Internal Medicine* 138 (2003): 430–431.

Fairfield, K. M., and R. H. Fletcher. "Vitamins for chronic disease prevention in adults: Scientific review." *Journal of the American Medical Association* 287 (2002): 3116–3126.

Fletcher, R. H., and K. M. Fairfield. "Vitamins for chronic disease prevention in adults: Clinical applications." *Journal of the American Medical Association* 287 (2002): 3127–3129.

Frei, B. "Efficacy of dietary antioxidants to prevent oxidative damage and inhibit chronic disease." *Journal of Nutrition* 134 (2004): 3196S–3198S.

Hathcock, J. N. et al. "Vitamins E and C are safe across a broad range of intakes." *American Journal of Clinical Nutrition* 81 (2005): 736–745.

McKully, K. S. *The Homocysteine Revolution.* Keats Publishing, 1997.

Oakley, G. P. Jr., editorial. "Eat right and take a multivitamin." *New England Journal of Medicine* 338 (1998): 1060–1061.

Plotnick, G. D.; M. C. Corretti; and R. A. Vogel. "Effect of antioxidant vitamins on the transient impairment of endothelium dependent brachial artery vasoactivity following a single high-fat meal." *Journal of the American Medical Association* 278 (1997): 1682–1686.

Tansey, W. P. "Death, destruction, and the proteasome." *New England Journal of Medicine* 351 (2004): 393–394.

Warnholtz, A. et al. "Antioxidants and endothelial dysfunction in hyperlipidemia." *Current Hypertension Reports* 3 (2001): 53–60.

VITAMIN C
Block, G. "Vitamin C and cancer prevention: The epidemiologic evidence." *American Journal of Clinical Nutrition.* Suppl. no. 53 (1991): 270S–282S.

Carpenter, K. J. *The History of Scurvy and Vitamin C.* Cambridge University Press, 1986.

Carr, A. C., and B. Frei. "Toward a new recommended dietary allowance for vitamin C based on antioxidant and health effects in humans." *American Journal of Clinical Nutrition* 69 (1999): 1086–1078.

Heitzer, T. et al. "Antioxidant vitamin C improves endothelial dysfunction in chronic smokers." *Circulation* 94 (1996): 6–9.

Jacques, P. F. et al. "Long-term vitamin C supplement use and prevalence of early age-related lens opacities." *American Journal of Clinical Nutrition* 66 (1997): 911–916.

Levine, G. N. et al. "Ascorbic acid reverses endothelial vasomototor dysfunction in patients with coronary artery disease." *Circulation* 93 (1996): 1107–1113.

Osganian, S. K. et al. "Vitamin C and risk of coronary heart disease in women." *Journal of the American College of Cardiology* 42 (2003): 246–252.

Perticone, F. et al. "Obesity and body fat distribution induce endothelial dysfunction by oxidative stress: Protective effect of vitamin C." *Diabetes* 50 (2001): 159–165.

Price, K. D.; C. S. Price; and R. D. Reynolds. "Hyperglycemia-induced ascorbic acid deficiency promotes endothelial dysfunction and the development of atherosclerosis." *Atherosclerosis* 158 (2001): 1–12.

Silvestro, A. et al. "Vitamin C prevents endothelial dysfunction induced by acute exercise in patients with intermittent claudication." *Atherosclerosis* 165 (2002): 277–283.

Solzbach, U. et al. "Vitamin C improves endothelial dysfunction of epicardial coronary arteries in hypertensive patients." *Circulation* 96 (1997): 1513–1519.

Taddei, S. et al. "Vitamin C improves endothelium-dependent vasodilation by restoring nitric oxide activity in essential hypertension." *Circulation* 97 (1998): 2222–2229.

Timimi, F. K. et al. "Vitamin C improves endothelium-dependent vasodilation in patients with insulin-dependent diabetes mellitus." *Journal of the American College of Cardiology* 31 (1998): 552–557.

Valero, M. P. et al. "Vitamin C is associated with reduced risk of cataract in a Mediterranean population." *Journal of Nutrition* 132 (2002): 1299–1306.

VITAMIN E

Engler, M. M. et al. "Antioxidant vitamins C and E improve endothelial function in children with hyperlipidemia: Endothelial assessment of risk from lipids in youth (EARLY) trial." *Circulation* 108 (2003): e9016–e9017.

GISSI-Prevenzione Investigators. "Dietary supplementation with n-3 polyunsaturated fatty acids and vitamin E after myocardial infarction: Results of the GISSI-Prevenzione trial." *Lancet* 354 (1999): 447–455.

Graat, J. M.; E. G. Schouten; and F. J. Kok. "Effect of daily vitamin E and multivitamin-mineral supplementation on acute respiratory tract infections in elderly persons: A randomized controlled trial." *Journal of the American Medical Association* 228 (2002): 715–721.

Jacques, P. F. et al. "Long-term nutrient intake and 5-Year change in nuclear lens opacities." *Archives of Ophthalmology* 123 (2005): 517–526.

Meydani, S. N. et al. "Vitamin E supplementation and in vivo immune response in healthy elderly subjects: A randomized controlled trial." *Journal of the American Medical Association* 227 (1997): 1380–1386.

Miller, E. R. III et al. "Meta-analysis: High-dosage vitamin E supplementation may increase all-cause mortality." *Annals of Internal Medicine* 145 (2005): 37–46.

Packer, L. et al. "Future directions in clinical vitamin E research: Panel discussion B." *Annals of the New York Academy of Sciences* 1031 (2004): 313–323.

Rimm, E. B. et al. "Vitamin E consumption and the risk of coronary heart disease in men." *New England Journal of Medicine* 328 (1993): 1450–1456.

Stampfer, M. J. et al. "Vitamin E consumption and the risk of coronary disease in women." *New England Journal of Medicine* 328 (1993): 1444–1449.

Stephens, N. G. et al. "Randomised controlled trial of vitamin E in patients with coronary disease: Cambridge Heart Antioxidant Study (CHAOS)." *Lancet* 347 (1996): 781–786.

Taub, Edward A., M.D., editorial response. "Eat an apple a day and take your vitamins." *Annals Online* (2004): http://www.annals.org/cgi/eletters/142/1/37#707.

Traber, M. G., and L. Packer. "Vitamin E: Beyond antioxidant function." *American Journal of Clinical Nutrition* Suppl. no. 6 (1996): 1501S-1509S.

Yusuf, S. et al. "Vitamin E supplementation and cardiovascular events in high-risk patients." *New England Journal of Medicine* 342 (2000): 154–160.

COENZYME Q10

Bagchi, D. "Coenzyme Q10: A novel cardiac antioxidant." *Journal of Orthomolecular Medicine* 12 (1997): 4–10.

Bargossi, A. M. et al. "Exogenous CoQlO supplementation prevents plasma ubiquinone reduction induced by HMG-CoA reductase inhibitors." *Molecular Aspects of Medicine* Suppl. no. 15 (2004): S187–S193.

Burke, B. E. "Randomized, double blind, placebo-controlled trial of CoQ10 in isolated systolic hypertension." *Southern Medical Journal* 94 (2001): 1112–1117.

Greenberg, S., and W. Frishman. "Coenzyme Q10: A new drug for cardiovascular disease." *Journal of Clinical Pharmacology* 30 (1990): 596–608.

Hofman-Bang, C. "Coenzyme Q10 as an adjunctive treatment of congestive heart failure." *American College of Cardiology* 19 (1992): 216A.

Langsjoen, P., and A. Langsjoen. "Overview of the use of CoQ10 in cardiovascular disease." *BioFactors* 9 (1999): 273–284.

Langsjoen, P. et al." A six-year clinical study of therapy of cardiomyopathy with coenzyme Q10." *International Journal of Tissue Reactions* 12 (1990): 169–171.

Mohr, D. et al. "Dietary supplementation with coenzyme Q10 results in increased levels of ubiquinol-10." *Biochim Biophys Acta* 1126 (1992): 247–254.

Morisco, C., and B. Trimarco. "Effect of coenzyme Q10 therapy in patients with congestive heart failure: A long-term multicenter randomized study." *Clinical Investigation* 71 (1993): S134–S136.

Overvad, K. et al. "Coenzyme Q10 in health and disease." *European Journal of Clinical Nutrition* 53 (1999): 764–770.

Sarter, B. "Coenzyme Q10 and cardiovascular disease: A review." *Journal of Cardiovascular Nursing* 16 (2002): 9–20.

Singh, R. B. et al. "Coenzyme Q10 and its role in heart disease." *Journal of Clinical Biochemistry Nutrition* 26 (1999): 109–118.

Soja, A. M., and S. A. Mortensen. "Treatment of congestive heart failure with CoQ10, illuminated by meta-analyses of clinical trials." *Molecular Aspects of Medicine* 18 (1997): S159–S168.

Tatjana, R. et al. "Atorvastatin decreases the coenzyme Q10 level in the blood of patients at risk for cardiovascular disease and stroke." *Archives of Neurology* 61 (2004): 889–892.

VITAMIN D

Bischoff-Ferrari, H. A. et al. "Estimation of optimal serum concentrations of 25- hydroxyvitamin D for multiple health outcomes." *American Journal of Clinical Nutrition* 84 (2006): 18–28.

Campbell, M. J., and H. P. Koeffler. "Toward therapeutic intervention of cancer by vitamin D compounds." *Journal of the National Cancer Institute* 89 (1997): 182–85.

Dawson-Hughes, B. et al. "Effect of calcium and vitamin D supplementation on bone density in men and women 65 years of age or older." *New England Journal of Medicine* 337 (1997): 670–676.

Gloth, F. M. III et al. "Vitamin D deficiency in homebound elderly persons." *Journal of the American Medical Association* 274 (1995): 1683–1686.

Grau, M. V. et al. "Vitamin D, calcium supplementation, and colorectal adenomas: Results of a randomized trial." *Journal of the National Cancer Institute* 5 (2003): 1765–1771.

LeBoff, M. S. et al. "Occult vitamin D deficiency in postmenopausal U.S. women with acute hip fracture." *Journal of the American Medical Association* 281 (1999): 1505–1509.

Skinner, H. et al. "Vitamin D intake and the risk for pancreatic cancer in two cohort studies." *Cancer Epidemiology Biomarkers & Prevention* 15 (2006): 1688–1695.

Thomas, M. K. et al. "Hypovitaminosis D in medical inpatients." *New England Journal of Medicine* 338 (1998): 777–783.

Utiger, R. D. "The need for more vitamin D." *New England Journal of Medicine* 338 (1998): 828–829.

FISH OIL (OMEGA-3 FATTY ACIDS)

American Heart Association Scientific Statement. "Fish consumption, fish oil, omega-3 fatty acids, and cardiovascular disease." *Circulation* 106 (2002): 2747.

Albert, C. M.; H. Campos; M. J. Stampfer et al. "Blood levels of long-chain n-3 fatty acids and the risk of sudden death." *New England Journal of Medicine* 346 (2002): 1113–1118.

Chin, J. P., and A. M. Dart. "How do fish oils affect vascular function?" *Clinical and Experiment Pharmacology Physiology* 22 (1995): 71–81.

Darlington, L. G., and T. W. Stone. "Antioxidants and fatty acids in the amelioration of rheumatoid arthritis and related disorders." *British Journal of Nutrition* 85 (2001): 251–269.

Das, U. N. "Long-chain polyunsaturated fatty acids interact with nitric oxide, superoxide anion, and transforming growth factor-beta to prevent human essential hypertension." *European Journal of Clinical Nutrition* 58 (2004): 195–203.

Daviglus, M. L. et al. "Fish consumption and the 30-year risk of fatal myocardial infarction." *New England Journal of Medicine* 336 (1997): 1046–1053.

De Lorgeril, M. et al. "Mediterranean diet, traditional risk factors, and the rate of cardiovascular complications after myocardial infarction: Final report of the Lyon Diet Heart Study." *Circulation* 99 (1999): 779–785.

GISSI-Prevenzione Investigators. "Dietary supplementation with n-3 polyunsaturated fatty acids and vitamin E after myocardial infarction: Results of the GISSI-Prevenzione trial." *Lancet* 354 (1999): 447–455.

Harris, W. S.; Y. Park; and W. L. Isley. "Cardiovascular disease and long-chain omega-3 fatty acids." *Current Opinions Lipidology* 14 (2003): 9–14.

Hu, F. B. et al. "Fish and omega-3 fatty acid intake and risk of coronary heart disease in women." *Journal of the American Medical Association* 287 (2002): 1815–1821.

Kris-Etherton, P. M. et al. "Omega-3 fatty acids and cardiovascular disease: New recommendations from the American Heart Association." *Arteriosclerosis, Thrombosis and Vascular Biology* 23 (2003): 151–152.

Kromhout, D. et al. "The inverse relation between fish consumption and 20-year mortality from coronary heart disease." *New England Journal of Medicine* 312 (1985): 1205–1209.

Laidlaw, M., and B. J. Holub. "Effects of supplementation with fish oil-derived n-3 fatty acids and y-linolenic acid on circulating plasma lipids and fatty acid profiles in women." *American Journal of Clinical Nutrition* 77 (2003): 37–42.

McVeigh, G. E. et al. "Fish oil improves arterial compliance in non-insulin–dependent diabetes mellitus." *Arteriosclerosis, Thrombosis and Vascular Biology* 14 (1994): 1425–1429.

Oh, K. et al. "Dietary fat intake and risk of coronary heart disease in women: 20 years of follow-up of the Nurses' Health Study." *American Journal of Epidemiology* 161 (2005): 672–679.

Simopoulos, A. P. "Essential fatty acids in health and chronic disease." *American Journal of Clinical Nutrition* 70 (1999): 560S–569S.

Stoll, A. *The Omega Connection.* Simon and Schuster, 2001.

FOLIC ACID AND B VITAMINS

Baik, H. W., and R. M. Russell. "Vitamin B12 deficiency in the elderly." *Annual Review of Nutrition* 19 (1999): 357–377.

Botto, L. D. et al. "Neural-tube defects." *New England Journal of Medicine* 341 (1999): 1509–1519.

Br nstrup, A. et al. "Effects of folic acid and combination of folic acid and vitamins B-12 on plasma homocysteine concentrations in healthy, young women." *American Journal of Clinical Nutrition* 68 (1998): 1104–1110.

Chambers, J. C. et al. "Improved vascular endothelial function after oral B vitamins: An effect mediated through reduced concentrations of free plasma homocysteine." *Circulation* 102 (2000): 2479–2483.

Clarke, R. et al. "Hyperhomocysteinemia: An independent risk factor for vascular disease." *New England Journal of Medicine* 324 (1999): 1149–1155.

Das, U. "Folic acid says NO to vascular disease." *Nutrition* 19 (2003): 686–692.

Doshi, S. N. "Folate improves endothelial function in coronary artery disease." *Arteriosclerosis, Thrombosis and Vascular Biology* 21 (2001): 1196–1202.

Giovannucci, E. "Multivitamin use, folate and colon cancer in women in the Nurses' Health Study." *Annals of Internal Medicine* 129 (1998): 517–524.

Kim, Y. I. "Folate and cancer prevention: A new medical application of folate beyond hyperhomocysteinemia and neural tube defects." *Nutr Rev* 57 (1999): 314–321.

Lobo, A. et al. "Reduction of homocysteine levels in coronary artery disease by low-dose folic acid combined with vitamins B6 and B12." *American Journal of Cardiology* 83 (1999): 821–825.

Milunsky, A. et al. "Multivitamin/folic acid supplementation in early pregnancy reduces the prevalence of neural tube defects." *Journal of the American Medical Association* 262 (1989): 2847–2852.

Naurath, H. J. et al. "Effects of vitamin B12, folate, and vitamin B6 supplements in elderly people with normal serum vitamin concentrations." *Lancet* 346 (1995): 85–89.

Nygard, O. et al. "Major lifestyle determinants of plasma total homocysteine distribution: The Hordaland Homocysteine Study." *Am J Clin Nutr* 67 (1998): 263–270.

Rimm, E. B. et al. "Folate and vitamin B6 from diet and supplements in relation to risk of coronary heart disease among women." *Journal of the American Medical Association* 279 (1998): 359–364.

Rohan, T. E. et al. "Dietary folate consumption and breast cancer risk." *Journal of the National Cancer Institute* 92 (2000): 266–269.

Shaw, G. M. et al. "Risks of orofacial clefts in children of women using multivitamins containing folic acid periconceptionally." *Lancet* 346 (1995): 393–396.

Su, L. J., and L. Arab. "Nutritional status of folate and colon cancer risk: Evidence from NHANES I epidemiologic follow-up study." *Annals of Epidemiology* 11 (2001): 65–72.

Verhaar, M. C. et al. "Effects of oral folic acid supplementation on endothelial function in familial hypercholesterolemia." *Circulation* 100 (1999): 335–338.

Welch, G. N., and J. Loscalzo. "Homocysteine and atherothrombosis." *New England Journal of Medicine* 338 (1998): 1042–1050.

Zhang, S. et al. "A prospective study of folate intake and the risk of breast cancer." *Journal of the American Medical Association* 281 (1999): 1632–1637.

L-ARGININE

Blum, A. et al. "Oral L-arginine in patients with coronary artery disease on medical management." *Circulation* 101 (2000): 2160–2164.

Boger, R. H. et al. "Restoring vascular nitric oxide formation by L-arginine improves the symptoms of intermittent claudication in patients with peripheral arterial occlusive disease." *Journal of the American College of Cardiology* 32 (1998): 1336–1344.

Ceremuzynski, I. et al. "Effect of supplemental oral L-arginine on exercise capacity in patients with stable angina pectoris." *American Journal of Cardiology* 80 (1997): 331–333.

Clarkson, P. et al. "Oral L-arginine improves endothelium-dependent dilation in hypercholesterolemic young adults." *Journal of Clinical Investigation* 97 (1996): 1989–1994.

Schulman, S. P. et al. "L-arginine therapy in acute myocardial infarction: The vascular interaction with age in myocardial infarction (VINTAGE MI) randomized clinical trial." *Journal of the American Medical Association* 295 (2006): 58–64.

VITAMIN A

Feskanich, D. et al. "Vitamin A intake and hip fractures among postmenopausal women." *Journal of the American Medical Association* 287 (2002): 47–54.

Lips, P., editorial. "Hypervitaminosis A and fractures." *New England Journal of Medicine* 348 (2003): 347–349.

Michaelsson, K. et al. "Serum retinol levels and the risk of fracture." *New England Journal of Medicine* 348 (2003): 287–294.

Penninston, K. L., and S. A. Tanumihardjo. "The acute and toxic affects of vitamin A." *American Journal of Clinical Nutrition* 83 (2006): 191–201.

HEALTHY NUTRITION

Albert, C. M. et al. "Fish consumption and risk of sudden cardiac death." *Journal of the American Medical Association* 279 (1998): 23–28.

Anderson, J. W. et al. "Meta-analysis of the effects of soy protein intake on serum lipids." *New England Journal of Medicine* 333 (1995): 276–282.

Anderson, R. A. et al. "Is the fat meal a trigger for acute coronary syndromes?" *Atherosclerosis* 159 (2001): 9–15.

Bae, J. H. et al. "Postprandial hypertriglyceridemia impairs endothelial function by enhanced oxidant stress." *Atherosclerosis* 155 (2001): 517–523.

de Lorgeril, M. et al. "Mediterranean diet, traditional risk factors, and the rate of cardiovascular complications after myocardial infarction: Final report of the Lyon Diet Heart Study." *Circulation* 99 (1999): 779–785.

Esposito, K. et al. "Effect of a Mediterranean-style diet on endothelial dysfunction and markers of vascular inflammation in the metabolic syndrome: A randomized trial." *Journal of the American Medical Association* 292 (2004): 1440–1446.

Hu, F. B. et al. "Nut consumption and risk of coronary heart disease: A review of epidemiologic evidence." *Current Atherosclerosis Reports* 1(1999): 204–209.

———. "Dietary fat intake and the risk of coronary heart disease in women." *New England Journal of Medicine* 337 (1997): 1491–1499.

———. "The Mediterranean diet and mortality—olive oil and beyond." *New England Journal of Medicine* 348 (2003): 2595–2596.

Jenkins, D. J. A. et al, editorial. "Diet and cholesterol reduction." *Annals of Internal Medicine* 142 (2005): 793–795.

———. "Effects of a dietary portfolio of cholesterol-lowering foods vs lovastatin on serum lipids and C-reactive protein." *Journal of the American Medical Association* 290 (2003): 502–510.

Kim, T. B. et al. "Mediterranean diet, lifestyle factors, and 10-year mortality in elderly European men and women: The HALE Project." *Journal of the American Medical Association* 292 (2004): 1433–1439.

Kris-Etherton, P. et al. "Lyon Diet Heart Study: Benefits of a Mediterranean-style, national cholesterol education program/American Heart Association step I dietary pattern on cardiovascular disease." *Circulation* 103 (2001): 1823–1825.

Leaf, A., editorial. "Dietary prevention of coronary heart disease: The Lyon Diet Heart Study." *Circulation* (1999): 733–735.

Levine, G. et al. "Cholesterol reduction in cardiovascular disease." *New England Journal of Medicine* 332 (1995): 512–521.

Nestle, M. "Mediterranean diets: Historical and research overview." *American Journal of Clinical Nutrition* 61 (1995): 1313S–1320S.

Nicholls, S. et al. "Consumption of saturated fat impairs the anti-inflammatory properties of high-density lipoproteins and endothelial function." *Journal of the American College of Cardiology* 48 (2006): 715–720.

Rimm, E. B., and M. J. Stampfer, editorial. "Diet, lifestyle, and longevity—the next steps?" *Journal of the American Medical Association* 292 (2004): 1490–1492.

Trichopoulou, A., and P. Lagiou. "Healthy traditional Mediterranean diet: An expression of culture, history and lifestyle." *Nutrition Review* 55 (1997): 383–389.

Vogel, R. et al. "Effect of a single high-fat meal on endothelial function in healthy subjects." *The American Journal of Cardiology* 79 (1997): 350–354.

———. "The postprandial effect of components of the Mediterranean diet on endothelial function." *Journal of the American College of Cardiology* 36 (2000): 1455–1460.

Willett, W. et al. "Mediterranean diet pyramid: A cultural model for healthy eating." *American Journal of Clinical Nutrition* 61 (1995): 1402–1406.

Williams, M. et al. "Impaired endothelial function following a meal rich in used cooking fat." *Journal of the American College of Cardiology* 33 (1999): 1050–1055.

Wolk, A. et al. "Long-term intake of dietary fiber and decreased risk of coronary heart disease among women." *Journal of the American Medical Association* 281 (1999): 1998–2004.

WEIGHT MANAGEMENT

Baik, I. et al. "Adiposity and mortality in men." *American Journal of Epidemiology* 152 (2000): 264–271.

Brody, J. "Personal Health: Forget the Second Helpings. It's the First Ones That Supersize Your Waistline." *New York Times,* July 11, 2006.

Caballero, A. "Endothelial Dysfunction in obesity and insulin resistance: A road to diabetes and heart disease." *Obesity Research* 11 (2003): 1278–1289.

Esposito, K. et al. "Effect of lifestyle changes on erectile dysfunction in obese men: A randomized controlled trial." *Journal of the American Medical Association* 291 (2004): 2978—2984.

Fraser. L. *Losing It: America's Obsession with Weight and an Industry that Feeds on It.* Dutton Publishers, 1997.

Huang, P. L., editorial, "Unraveling the links between diabetes, obesity, and cardiovascular disease." *Circulation Research* 96 (2005): 1129.

Kassirer, J. P., and M. Angell. "Losing weight—an ill-fated new year's resolution." *New England Journal of Medicine* 338 (1998): 52–54.

Klem, M. L. et al. "Patterns of weight loss maintenance." *The American Journal of Clinical Nutrition* 66 (1997): 239–246.

Lee, I. M. et al. "Body weight and mortality: A 27-year follow-up of middle-aged men." *Journal of the American Medical Association* 270 (1993): 2823–2828.

Manson, J. E. et al. "Body weight and mortality among women." *New England Journal of Medicine* 333 (1995): 677–685.

National Task Force on the Prevention and Treatment of Obesity. "Overweight, obesity, and health risk." *Archives of Internal Medicine* 160 (2000): 898–904.

Nestle, M., and M. Jacobson. "Halting the obesity epidemic: A public health policy approach." *Public Health Reports* 115 (2000): 12–24.

Pescatello, L. et al. "Physical activity mediates a healthier body weight in the presence of obesity." *British Journal of Sports Medicine* 34 (2000): 86–93.

Saigal, C. S. "Obesity and erectile dysfunction: Common problems, common solution?" *Journal of the American Medical Association* 291 (2004): 3011–3012.

Sciacqua, A. et al. "Weight loss in combination with physical activity improves endothelial dysfunction in human obesity." *Diabetes Care* 26 (2003): 1673–1678.

Singhal, A. "Endothelial dysfunction: Role in obesity-related disorders and the early origins of CVD." *Proceedings of the Nutrition Society* 64 (2005): 15–22.

Steinberger, J. et al. "Adiposity in childhood predicts obesity and insulin resistance in young adulthood." *Journal of Pediatrics* 138 (2001): 469–473.

Wildman, R. P. et al. "Measures of obesity are associated with vascular stiffness in young and older adults." *Hypertension* 42 (2003): 468–473.

Willett, W. et al. "Guidelines for healthy weight." *New England Journal of Medicine* 341 (1999): 427–434.

Williams, I. L. et al. "Obesity, atherosclerosis and the vascular endothelium: Mechanisms of reduced nitric oxide bioavailability in obese humans." *International Journal of Obesity* 26 (2002): 754–764.

Williamson, D., editorial. "The prevention of obesity." *New England Journal of Medicine* 341 (1999): 1140–1141.

Wing, R. R., and J. O. Hill. "Successful weight loss maintenance." *Annual Review of Nutrition* 21 (2001): 323–341.

EXERCISE

Gill, J. M. R. et al. "Effects of prior moderate exercise on postprandial metabolism and vascular function in lean and centrally obese men." *Journal of the American College of Cardiology* 44 (2004): 2375–2382.

Hambrecht, R. "Effect of exercise on coronary endothelial function in patients with coronary artery disease." *New England Journal of Medicine* 342 (2002): 454-460.

Hambrecht, R. et al. "Regular physical exercise corrects endothelial dysfunction and improves exercise capacity in patients with chronic heart failure." *Circulation* 24 (1998): 2709–2715.

Hornig, B. et al. "Physical training improves endothelial function in patients with chronic heart failure." *Circulation* 93 (1996): 210–214.

Hu, F. B. et al. "Adiposity compared with physical activity in predicting mortality among women." *New England Journal of Medicine* 351 (2004): 2694–2703.

Jungersten, L. et al. "Both physical fitness and acute exercise regulate nitric oxide formation in healthy humans." *Journal of Applied Physiology* 82 (1997): 760–764.

Lee, I. M. et al. "Physical activity and coronary heart disease in women: Is 'no pain, no gain' passé?" *Journal of the American Medical Association* 285 (2001): 1447–1454.

Lili, J. I. "Exercise-induced modulation of antioxidant defense." *Annals New York Academy of Sciences* 959 (2002): 82–92.

Manson, J. E. et al. "Walking compared with vigorous exercise for the prevention of cardiovascular events in women." *New England Journal of Medicine* 347 (2002): 716–725.

Padilla, J. et al. "The effect of acute exercise on endothelial function following a high-fat meal." *European Journal of Applied Physiology* 98 (2006): 256–262.

Paganini-Hill, A. et al. "Exercise and other risk factors in the prevention of hip fracture: The Leisure World Study." *Epidemiology* 2 (1991): 16–25.

Roberts, C. K. et al. "Effect of diet and exercise intervention on blood pressure, insulin, oxidative stress, and nitric oxide availability." *Circulation* 106 (2002): 2530–2532.

Shephard, R. J., and Balady, G. J. "Exercise as cardiovascular therapy." *Circulation* 99 (1999): 963–972.

Stefanick, M. et al. "Effects of diet and exercise in men and postmenopausal women with low levels of HDL cholesterol and high levels of LDL cholesterol." *New England Journal of Medicine* 339 (1998): 12–20.

Taddei, S. et al. "Physical activity prevents age-related impairment in nitric oxide availability in elderly athletes." *Circulation* 101 (2000): 2896–2901.

Tune, I. et al. "Physical activity and the risk of breast cancer." *New England Journal of Medicine* 336 (1997): 1269–1275.

Vita, J. A. and J. F. Keaney Jr., editorial. "Exercise—toning up the endothelium." *New England Journal of Medicine* 342 (2000): 503–505.

ADDICTIONS

Ambrose, A., and R. S. Barua. "The pathophysiology of cigarette smoking and cardio-vascular disease: An update." *Journal of the American College of Cardiology* 43 (2004): 1731–1737.

Barnoya, J., and S. A. Glantz. "Cardiovascular effects of secondhand smoke: Nearly as large as smoking." *Circulation* 111 (2005): 2684–2698.

Beck, A. T. *Cognitive Therapy of Substance Abuse.* Guilford, 1993.

Black C. E. et al. "Acute effects of cigarette smoke on inflammation and oxidative stress: A review." *Thorax* 59 (2004): 713–721.

Bradshaw, J. *Healing the Shame that Binds You.* HCI Books, 1998.

Giovannucci, E. et al. "Alcohol, low-methionine–low-folate diets, and risk of colon cancer in men." *Journal of the National Cancer Institute* 87 (1995): 265–273.

Goldberg, I. J. et al. "Wine and your heart: A science advisory for healthcare profes-sionals from the nutrition committee, council on epidemiology and prevention, and council on cardiovascular nursing of the American Heart Association." *Circulation* 103 (2001): 472–475.

Klatsky, A. L. et al. "The relationships between alcoholic beverage use and other traits to blood pressure: A new Kaiser Permanente study." *Circulation* 73 (1986): 628–636.

Masahiko, T. M. et al. "Smoking a single cigarette rapidly reduces combined concen-trations of nitrate and nitrite and concentrations of antioxidants in plasma." *Circulation.* 105 (2002): 1155–1157.

National Institute on Drug Abuse Research Report Series. *Tobacco Addiction* (2006), http://www.nida.nih.gov/researchreports/nicotine/Nicotine.html.

Neunteufl, T. "Contribution of nicotine to acute endothelial dysfunction in long-term smokers." *Journal of the American College of Cardiology* 39 (2002): 251–256.

Prochaska, J. O. *Changing for Good.* Avon, 1994.

Pursch, J. A. *Dear Doc: The Noted Authority Answers Your Questions on Drinking and Drugs.* Compcare Publications, 1985.

Raupach, T. "Secondhand smoke as an acute threat for the cardiovascular system: A change in paradigm." *European Heart Journal* 27 (2006): 386–392.

Saitz, R. "Unhealthy alcohol use." *New England Journal of Medicine* 352 (2005): 596–607.

Smith-Warner, S. A. et al. "Alcohol and breast cancer in women." *Journal of the Amer-ican Medical Association* 279 (1998): 535–540.

Taub, Edward A., M.D. *How to Quit: The American Medical Association National Wellness Stop Smoking Campaign.* Orbis Broadcast Group, 1994.

———. *The Wellness Rx.* Prentice Hall, 1995.

van der Vaart, H. et al. "Acute effects of cigarette smoke on inflammation and oxidative stress: A review." *Thorax* 59 (2004): 713–721.

Vleeming, W. et al. "The role of nitric oxide in cigarette smoking and nicotine addic-tion." *Nicotine Tobacco Research* 4 (2002): 341–348.

Witteman, J. C. et al. "Relation of moderate alcohol consumption and the risk of systemic hypertension in women." *American Journal of Cardiology* 65 (1990): 633–637.

NO AND STRESS

Benson, H. "The physiology of meditation." *Scientific American* 226 (1972): 84–90.

Chrousos, G. P. "A healthy body in a healthy mind—and vice versa—the damaging power of uncontrollable stress." *Journal of Clinical Endocrinology and Metabolism* 83 (1998): 1842–1845.

———. "Stress, chronic inflammation, and emotional and physical well-being: Concurrent effects and chronic sequelae." *Journal of Allergy and Clinical Immunology* 106 (2000): 275–291.

Dawson, T. M., and S. H. Snyder. "Gases as biological messengers: Nitric oxide and carbon monoxide in the brain." *Journal of Neuroscience* 14 (1994): 5147–5159.

Elenkov, I. J. et al. "The sympathetic nerve—an integrative interface between two supersystems: The brain and the immune system." *Pharmacological Reviews* 52 (2000): 595–638.

Esch, T. et al. "Stress-related diseases-a potential role for nitric oxide." *Medical Science Monitor* 8 (2002): RA 103–118.

González-Albo, M. C. "The human temporal cortex: Characterization of neurons expressing nitric oxide synthase, neuropeptides and calcium-binding proteins." *Cerebral Cortex* 11 (2001): 1170–1181.

Harris, K. et al. "Associations between psychological traits and endothelial function in postmenopausal women." *Psychosomatic Medicine* 65 (2003): 402–409.

———. "Interactions between autonomic nervous system activity and endothelial function: A model for the development of cardiovascular disease." *Psychosomatic Medicine* 66 (2004): 153–164.

Kara, P., and M. J. Friedlander. "Dynamic modulation of cerebral cortex synaptic function by nitric oxide." *Progress in Brain Research* 118 (1998): 183–198.

Kutz, I.; J. Z. Borysenko; and H. Benson. "Meditation and psychotherapy: A rationale for the integration of dynamic psychotherapy, the relaxation response and mindfulness meditation." *American Journal of Psychiatry* 142 (1985): 1–8.

Jayasinghe, S. R. "Yoga in cardiac health." *European Journal of Cardiovascular Prevention and Rehabilitation* 11 (2004): 369–375.

Lucini, D. et al. "Impact of chronic psychosocial stress on autonomic cardiovascular regulation in otherwise healthy subjects." *Hypertension* 46 (2005): 1201–1206.

McEwen, B. S. "Protective and damaging effects of stress mediators." *New England Journal of Medicine* 338 (1998): 171–179.

Moreno-Lopez, B., and D. Gonzalez-Forero. "Nitric oxide and synaptic dynamics in the adult brain: Physiopathological aspects." *Review Neurosciences* 17 (2006): 309–357.

Moroz, L. L. "Gaseous transmission across time and species." *American Zoologist* 41 (2001): 304–320.

Ornish, D. "Can lifestyle changes reverse coronary artery disease?" *Lancet* 336 (1990): 129.

Rumsfeld, J. S., and M. P. Ho. "Depression and cardiovascular disease: A call for recognition." *Circulation* 111 (2005): 250–253.

Sherwood, A. et al. "Impaired endothelial function in coronary heart disease patients with depressive symptomatology." *Journal of the American College of Cardiology* 46 (2005): 656–659.

Sivasankaran, S. "The effect of a six-week yoga training and meditation program on endothelial function." *American Heart Association Scientific Sessions,* 2004.

Snyder, S. H. and Dawson, T. M. "Nitric oxide and related substances as neural messengers." *American College of Neuropsychopharmacology,* 2000, http://www.acnp.org/g4/GN401000060/60R.html.

Stefano, G. B. et al. "The placebo effect and the relaxation response: Neural processes and their coupling to constitutive nitric oxide." *Brain Research Reviews* 35 (2001): 1–19.

———. "The therapeutic use of the relaxation response in stress-related diseases." *Medical Science Monitor* 9 (2003): RA23–RA34.

Sternberg, E. M., and P. W. Gold. "The mind-body interaction in disease." *Scientific American, Special Edition: The Hidden Mind* 12 (2002): 82–29.

Vale, S. "Psychosocial stress and cardiovascular diseases." *Postgraduate Medicine Journal* 81 (2005): 429–435.

Vitetta, L. et al. "Mind-body medicine: Stress and its impact on overall health and longevity." *Annals of the New York Academy of Sciences* 1057 (2005): 492–505.

STRESS MANAGEMENT

Beck, Aaron T., M.D. *Cognitive Therapy and the Emotional Disorders.* Meridian, 1967.

Benson, Herbert, M.D. *The Relaxation Response.* Morrow, 1975.

Borysenko, Joan, Ph.D. *Minding the Body, Mending the Mind.* Addison-Wesley, 1987.

Covey, Stephen R. *The 7 Habits of Highly Effective People.* Simon and Schuster, 1989.

Damasio, Anthony, M.D. *Looking for Spinoza: Joy, Sorrow and the Feeling Brain.* Harcourt, 2003.

Dyer, Wayne W. *The Power of Intention.* Hay House, 2006.

Kabat-Zinn, Jon, Ph.D. *Wherever You Are, There You Are.* Hyperion, 1994.

Krystal, Phyllis. *Cutting the Ties that Bind.* Aura Books, 1982.

Peale, Norman Vincent. *Power of Positive Thinking.* Fawcett Books, 1987.

Robbins, Anthony. *Awaken the Giant Within.* Free Press, 1992.

Sarno, John E., M.D. *The Mind Body Prescription.* Warner Books, 1998.

Seligman, Martin E. P., Ph.D. *Learned Optimism.* Vintage Books, 2006.

Simonton, O.C., M.D. et al. *Getting Well Again.* J.P. Tarcher, 1978.

Taub, Edward A., M.D. *Balance Your Body, Balance Your Life.* Pocket Books, 1999.

———. *The Seven Steps to Self Healing.* DK Publishing, 1996.

A WHOLE NEW REALITY

Angell, Marcia, M.D. *The Truth About the Drug Companies: How They Deceive Us and What to Do About It.* Random House, 2004.

Braunwald, Eugene, M.D. "Shattuck Lecture: Cardiovascular medicine at the turn of the millennium: Triumphs, concerns, and opportunities." *New England Journal of Medicine* 337 (1997): 1360–1369.

Frist, William, M.D. "Shattuck Lecture: Health care in the 21st century." *New England Journal of Medicine* 352 (2005): 267–272.

Lown, Bernard, M.D. *The Lost Art of Healing.* Houghton Mifflin, 1996.

Lundberg, George, M.D. "The American Healthcare System in 2005: Parts 1–7." www.medscape.com.

Murad, Ferid, M.D., Ph.D. "Shattuck Lecture: Discovery of nitric oxide and cyclic GMP in cell signaling and their role in drug development." *New England Journal of Medicine* (Publication date, forthcoming).

WELLNESS THEOLOGY

Groopman, J. "God at the bedside." *New England Journal of Medicine* 350 (2004): 1176–1178.

Johnson, K. S. "The influence of spiritual beliefs and practices on the treatment preferences of African Americans: A review of the literature." *Journal of the American Geriatrics Society* 53 (2005): 711–719.

Karen, E. et al. "Are you at peace?: One item to probe spiritual concerns at the end of life." *Archives of Internal Medicine* 166 (2006): 101–105.

Koenig, H. G. "Religion, spirituality, and medicine: How are they related and what does it mean?" *Mayo Clinic Proceedings* 76 (2001): 1189–1191.

Koenig. H. G. et al. "Religiosity and remission of depression in medically ill older patients." *American Journal of Psychiatry* 155 (1998): 536–542.

Lo, B. et al. "Discussing religious and spiritual issues at the end of life: A practical guide for physicians." *Journal of the American Medical Association* 287 (2002): 749–754.

Lynn, J. "Serving patients who may die soon and their families: The role of hospice and other services." *Journal of the American Medical Association* 285 (2001): 925–932.

Monroe, M. H. et al. "Primary care physician preferences regarding spiritual behavior in medical practice." *Archives of Internal Medicine* 163 (2003): 2751–2756.

Post, S. G. et al. "Physicians and patient spirituality: Professional boundaries, competency, and ethics." *Annals of Internal Medicine* 132 (2000): 578–583.

Puchalski, C. M., "Spirituality and end-of-life care: A time for listening and caring." *Journal of Palliative Medicine* 5 (2002): 289–294.

Puchalski, C. M. and Al Romer. "Taking a spiritual history allows clinicians to understand patients more fully." *Journal of Palliative Medicine* 3 (2000): 129–137.

Stuart-Smith K. "Demystified . . . Nitric oxide." *Molecular Pathology* 55 (2002): 360–366.

Sulmasy, D. P. "Spiritual issues in the care of dying patients: It's okay between me and God." *Journal of the American Medical Association* 296 (2006): 1385–1392.

INFLAMMATION, OXIDATIVE STRESS, AND ENTROPY

Abrams, J. "C-reactive protein, inflammation, and coronary risk: An update." *Cardiology Clinics* 21 (2003): 327–331.

Bonetti, P. O. et al. "Endothelial dysfunction: A marker of atherosclerotic risk." *Arteriosclerosis, Thrombosis and Vascular Biology* 23 (2003): 168–175.

Buckley, C. D. et al. "Endothelial cells, fibroblasts and vasculitis." *Rheumatology* 44 (2005): 860–863.

Celermajer, D.S. et al. "Aging is associated with endothelial dysfunction in healthy men years before the age-related decline in women." *Journal of the American College of Cardiology* 24 (1994): 471–476.

Cooke, J. P., and V. J. Dzau. "Nitric oxide synthase: Role in the genesis of vascular disease." *Annual Review of Medicine* 48 (1997): 489–509.

Das, U. N. "Free radicals, cytokines and nitric oxide in cardiac failure and myocardial infarction." *Molecular and Cellular Biochemistry* 215 (2000): 145–152.

Ehrenstein, M. R., editorial. "Statins for atherosclerosis—as good as it gets?" *New England Journal of Medicine* 352 (2005): 73–75.

El-Magadmi, M. et al. "Systemic lupus erythematosus: An independent risk factor for endothelial dysfunction in women." *Circulation* 110 (2004): 399–404.

Goligorsky, G. S. et al. "Endothelial cell dysfunction leading to diabetic nephropathy: Focus on nitric oxide." *Hypertension* 37 (2001): 744–748.

Griffiths, M. J. et al. "Inhaled nitric oxide therapy in adults." *New England Journal of Medicine* 353 (2005): 2683–2695.

Hare, J. M., editorial. "Nitroso-redox balance in the cardiovascular system." *New England Journal of Medicine* 351 (2004): 2112–2114.

Heitzer, T. et al. "Endothelial dysfunction, oxidative stress, and risk of cardiovascular events in patients with coronary artery disease." *Circulation* 104 (2001): 2673–2678.

Kinlay, S., and P. Ganz. "Role of endothelial dysfunction in coronary artery disease and implications for therapy." *American Journal of Cardiology* 80 (1997): 11-I–16-I.

Koenig, W. "Inflammation and coronary heart disease: An overview." *Cardiology Review* 9 (2001): 31–35.

Mason, P. R. et al. "Nebivolol reduces nitroxidative stress and restores nitric oxide bioavailability in endothelium of black Americans." *Circulation* 112 (2005): 3795–3801.

Nathan, C. "Inflammation: Points of control." *Nature* 420 (2002): 846–852.

Nissen, S. E. et al. "Statin therapy, LDL cholesterol, C-reactive protein, and coronary artery disease." *New England Journal of Medicine* 352 (2005): 29–38.

Olshansky, S. J. et al. "A potential decline in life expectancy in the United States in the 21st century." *New England Journal of Medicine* 352 (2005): 1138–1145.

Preston, S. H., editorial. "Deadweight?—the influence of obesity on longevity." *New England Journal of Medicine* 352 (2005): 1135–1137.

Ramachandran, S. et al. "Biomarkers of cardiovascular disease: Molecular basis and practical considerations." *Circulation* 113 (2006): 2335–2362.

Ridker, P. M. et al. "C-reactive protein levels and outcomes after statin therapy." *New England Journal of Medicine* 352 (2005): 20–28.

Ross, R. "Atherosclerosis—an inflammatory disease." *New England Journal of Medicine* 340 (1999): 115–128.

Schreiber, M. D. et al. "Inhaled nitric oxide in premature infants with the respiratory distress syndrome." *New England Journal of Medicine* 349 (2003): 2099–2107.

Shah, S. H., and L. K. Newby. "C-reactive protein: A novel marker of cardiovascular risk." *Cardiology Review* 11 (2003): 169–179.

Stocker, R., and J. F. Keaney Jr. "Role of oxidative modifications in atherosclerosis." *Physiology Review* 84 (2004): 1381–1478.

Taylor, A. L. et al. "Combination of isosorbide dinitrate and hydralazine in African Americans with heart failure." *New England Journal of Medicine* 351 (2004): 2049–2057.

Thompson, I. M. et al. "Erectile dysfunction and subsequent cardiovascular disease." *Journal of the American Medical Association* 294 (2005): 2996–3002.

Tousoulis, D. et al. "Inflammatory and thrombotic mechanisms in coronary atherosclerosis." *Heart* 89 (2003): 993–997.

Vanhoutte, P. M. "Ageing and endothelial dysfunction." *European Heart Journal* Suppl 4 (2004): A8–A17.

Vaudo, G. et al. "Endothelial dysfunction in young patients with rheumatoid arthritis and low disease activity." *Annals of Rheumatoid Diseases* 63 (2004): 31–35.

Verma, S. et al. "C-reactive protein: Structure affects function." *Circulation* 109 (2004): 1914–1917.

———. "A self-fulfilling prophecy: C-reactive protein attenuates nitric oxide production and inhibits angiogenesis. Circulation 106 (2002): 913.

Wittstein, I. S. et al. "Neurohumoral features of myocardial stunning due to sudden emotional stress." *New England Journal of Medicine* 352 (2005): 539–548.

LAUGHTER AND MUSIC

Miller, M. "Divergent effects of laughter and mental stress on endothelial function: Potential impact of entertainment." (lecture, Scientific Session of the American College of Cardiology, March 6–9, 2005).

Salamon, E. et al. "Sound therapy induced relaxation: Down regulating stress processes and pathologies." *Medical Science Monitor* (2003).

Weitzberg, E. and J. O. Lundberg. "Humming greatly increases nasal nitric oxide." *American Journal of Respiratory and Critical Care Medicine* 166 (2002): 144–145.

CHOCOLATE AND WINE

Heiss, C. et al. "Endothelial function, nitric oxide, and cocoa flavanols." *Journal of Cardiovascular Pharmacology* 47 (2006): S128–S135.

Hermann, F. et al. "Dark chocolate improves endothelial and platelet function." *Heart* 92 (2006): 119–120.

Wallerath, T. et al. "Red wine increases the expression of human endothelial nitric oxide synthase: A mechanism that may contribute to its beneficial cardiovascular effects." *Journal of the American College of Cardiology* 41 (2003): 479–481.

INDEX

NOTES

NOTES

NOTES

NOTES

NOTES

NOTES